Principles of Reimbursement in Health Care

Donald F. Beck, M.B.A.

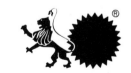

AN ASPEN PUBLICATION®
Aspen Systems Corporation
Rockville, Maryland
Royal Tunbridge Wells
1984

Library of Congress Cataloging in Publication Data

Beck, Donald F.
Principles of reimbursement in health care.

Includes index.
1. Hospitals—Finance 2. Insurance, Hospitalization.
3. Hospitals—Business management. 4. Medicare.
5. Hospitals—United States—Finance. 6. Insurance,
Hospitalization—United States. 7. Hospitals—United
States—Business management. I. Title. II. Title:
Reimbursement in health care.
[DNLM: 1. Reimbursement
mechanics. 2. Insurance, Health, Reimbursement.
3. Health insurance for aged and disabled, Title 18—
Economics 4. Medical assistance, Title 19—Economics.
5. Economics, Hospital—United States. WX 157 B393p]
RA971.3.B387   1983   362.1'1'0681   83-12300
ISBN: 0-89443-887-5

Publisher: John Marozsan
Editor-in-Chief: Michael Brown
Executive Managing Editor: Margot Raphael
Editorial Services: Ruth Judy
Printing and Manufacturing: Debbie Collins

Library of Congress Catalog Card Number: 83-12300
ISBN: 0-89443-887-5

Printed in the United States of America

2   3   4   5

To my wife
Andrea K. Beck

Table of Contents

Preface

Since the inception of Medicare and Medicaid in 1967, the health care industry has seen cost reimbursement become increasingly more restrictive. I have watched as hospital boards and administrators, seeing their financial base being eroded, sat back helplessly. Some have hired prestigious international firms or former intermediary auditors, believing that this will guarantee the maximum possible reimbursement. Consultants who specialize in reimbursement have reworked cost reports, obtaining millions of dollars in additional reimbursement under a contract in which they receive a percentage of the additional reimbursement. Although I do not work on a percentage basis, I have reworked cost reports prepared by experts and have obtained hundreds of thousands of additional dollars for hospitals.

True reimbursement experts agree that most hospitals are losing hundreds of thousands of dollars because of an inability to effectively manage cost reimbursement. It is clear that reimbursement must be managed throughout the year. Although millions of additional dollars are regained by firms specializing in cost report preparation, it is too late at year end to position the institution to take advantage of the most effective techniques. Reimbursement maximization is a year-round task. Aggressive for-profit chains recognize this and hire high-priced, full-time experts who are assigned a very small number of hospitals. These experts consider and report the reimbursement impact of every activity the hospital enters into throughout the year. Smaller chains and free-standing institutions are often at a disadvantage because of the mystique that surrounds reimbursement. This book was written to dispel this mystique.

Throughout the text hundreds of techniques and examples are presented. Every technique presented has been successfully used by a hospital somewhere in America. No one hospital has used all of these techniques. Indeed, it would be totally inappropriate to use all of the techniques in this book at one institution because the cost reports would lose their credibility. There is a distinct difference between being aggressive and giving up one's integrity. When there is a question on the appropriateness of a particular technique presented in this book for your institution, a competent professional should be consulted. If the institution can use a technique and still maintain its integrity, it should. If there is some reason to believe the technique is not appropriate for your institution, it should not be used. In making this determination it is important to remember that:

- Medicare and other cost reimbursement reports often depart from generally accepted accounting principles.
- Hundreds of techniques that were disallowed by Medicare and others have been upheld by the courts.
- Notwithstanding their good intentions, the intermediary and HCFA will think about a technique from a different point of view than that of the provider.

As this book was being completed, the laws governing Medicare reimbursement changed dramatically. However, hospitals are required to continue cost reporting through the transition from cost reimbursement to prospective reimbursement and for at least two years after full implementation of the new system (at least until the end of fiscal year 1988). Although cost will continue to be the dominant form of reimbursement for several years, major sections on diagnostic-related groups, prospective payment systems, TEFRA, and other new developments are included in the book, along with sections on Medicaid, Blue Cross, and other cost reports, and techniques dealing with rate review.

This is not a book on how to prepare cost reports. It is a book about managing reimbursement. It is hoped that this book will change the manner in which the reader thinks about reimbursement. Those who continue to believe that nothing can be done, that we must react but cannot act, probably will not survive. If this book changes the way in which you think about regulations, cost reports, rate setting, and financial management then it will have served its purpose.

I wish to express my appreciation to all those whose assistance and support made this book possible, especially to the reimbursement specialists throughout the country who have shared their ideas with me; to Penny Drain, who typed the manuscript, for her suggestions and patience; and finally to my wife, Andrea, for her support and encouragement.

Donald F. Beck

Chapter 1

Introduction

On July 30, 1965, the Congress of the United States established a program to provide health care for the aged. This program has significantly and permanently changed the delivery of health care in America. The Medicare program, Title 18, is part of the Social Security Amendments of 1965. Medicaid, Title 19 of the Social Security Act, provides grants to states for medical assistance programs.

THE MEDICARE PROGRAM

There were numerous government-sponsored health care programs in existence before 1965. However, none of these paralleled the scope of Medicare. Large-scale health insurance programs had been major political issues during several presidential campaigns prior to 1965. Both the Kennedy and Johnson administrations developed programs that eventually became the original Medicare program.

The Medicare program has two separate and distinct trusts. These are called Part A and Part B. The Part-A fund is financed by universal mandatory contributions through F.I.C.A. taxes. Part B provides a voluntary supplemental medical benefits plan. It was the original intent of Congress that Part A should reimburse hospitals and other providers of health care for reasonable costs. Part B was to reimburse hospitals and other institutional providers for reasonable costs and to reimburse physicians for usual and customary fees. Part B is optional and has a 20 percent coinsurance requirement.

Many of the regulations, forms, and calculations are necessary merely to separate the requirements of the two trust funds. This separation has proved to be expensive as well as counterproductive.

The secretary of the Department of Health and Human Services (HHS) (formerly Health, Education and Welfare) was given the authority to implement congressional law and intent through regulations. These regulations, if properly perfected by the secretary (see Chapter 3), have the force and effect of law. Therefore, it is important to note the effective dates of the regulations, which are published primarily in two government manuals. The first is Health Insurance Manual–10 (HIM-10), called the hospital manual. This manual outlines limits of coverage and Medicare billing practices. Health Insurance Manual–15 (HIM-15) is called the provider reimbursement manual. Part 1 of HIM-15 explains cost reporting rules and regulations. Part 2 provides copies of the current cost report forms and instructions for their use. These manuals, as well as regular updates, are available without charge from the intermediaries. Every hospital, nursing home, home health agency, and institutional provider should have current copies of both of these manuals and should keep them up to date. It should be noted that hospitals, nursing homes, and other providers are not bound by these manuals. However, they do simplify the application of Medicare principles.

THE MEDICAID PROGRAM

Public assistance for medical care has been administered by the states since 1950. This assistance has expanded, but the need for medical assistance has expanded at a greater pace. To satisfy the growing need, the Social Security Amendments of 1965 provided that, starting July 1, 1966, the federal government would provide grants to states for medical assistance. Medicaid is an optional program, but all of the states except Arizona have Medicaid programs at the time of this writing. In addition, Puerto Rico, Guam, and the Virgin Islands have Medicaid programs.

Medicaid provides medical assistance to persons because they are poor, aged, blind, or disabled. Medicaid recipients are called either categorically needy, because they fall into one of the applicable categories of assistance, or medically needy, because they lack sufficient funds to pay their medical bills.

Each of the 52 Medicaid programs is administered separately and funded by state as well as federal funds. Although each state can establish its own system for reimbursing hospitals, most Medicaid systems are geared to Medicare cost reimbursement principles.

In this book, we will address primarily the principles of Medicare in hospitals. Where applicable, techniques to maximize reimbursement from Medicaid cost reports, Blue Cross cost reports, and other reports are discussed. However, it is impossible in one volume to cover all 52 Medicaid plans and the numerous Blue Cross cost reports.

Although the narrative and illustrations are based primarily on short-term care hospitals, the principles discussed are applicable to home health agencies, nursing homes, skilled nursing facilities, and other providers of health care. Because Medicare principles and forms change frequently, specific line-by-line instructions are not presented in the text. The forms and instructions used at the time of this writing are included in Appendixes A through F.

THE COST REIMBURSEMENT PROCESS

History

The original intent of Congress was to pay a reasonable amount to hospitals for the care of Medicare patients. The wording in the original law stipulates that "nothing in this title shall be construed to authorize any Federal officer or employee . . . to exercise any supervision or control of any (health care) institution."[1] When Medicare and Medicaid began, this directive was followed. After a short time, however, the government regulations became more restrictive and demanding. There is still no mandated direct control over health care institutions, but the government substantially reduces payments to those institutions who do not comply. Today, there are entire volumes containing the complex set of regulations that interprets which provider costs Medicare and Medicaid recognize or allow.

Prudence and common sense are not principles of reimbursement. Like corporate income tax regulations, the Medicare regulations evolved to solve specific government problems or to stimulate specific objectives. If we think about what has happened in these programs, we can see that this was predictable. From the beginning, the Medicare program has exceeded its original budget. The Social Security Administration has never been given enough budget funds to pay for all of the required care, and they have had to use regulations to balance their budgets.

There are three important reasons why Medicare has consistently been underbudgeted:

1. Medicare, like Medicaid, has allowed the "worried well" to be hospitalized. There is not enough incentive built into these programs to keep the worried well from becoming hospitalized.
2. Medicare was initiated at a time when our country was undergoing a technology explosion as a result of the space program. This technology has had, and continues to have, a dramatic effect on health care

delivery. We are performing procedures now that were considered impossible a short time ago.

3. There has been a great increase in the number of physicians graduated each year from American medical colleges. In the late 1960s, the U.S. government offered grants and other incentives to states to create new medical schools, as well as to increase the size of existing medical schools. By 1975, the number of doctors graduating from American medical schools had doubled. Since physicians in this country create their own demand, as we increase the supply of physicians, we proportionately increase the demand for their services.

Other factors have contributed to the Medicare and Medicaid programs being greatly overbudget, but the three reasons cited above are the most important.

Many of the regulations and restrictions imposed upon providers were implemented as budget-balancing acts. In many instances, HHS is more restrictive than the government agency responsible for monitoring the area. This is appropriate when one considers the intent of Medicare regulations. For example, the Medicare regulations on pension plans, deferred compensation, and self-insurance are extraordinarily detailed. Medicare regulations do not always follow generally accepted accounting principles. For instance, the requirements on self-insurance malpractice funding impair the integrity of the financial statements. Nevertheless, they still must be followed for cost reporting purposes.

Medicare Cost Reports

The cost report is due on the last day of the third month following the close of the fiscal year. The intermediary can grant a 30-day extension but is not required to do this. However, there is no provision in the current regulations to withhold payments or to penalize the hospital until a cost report is more than 30 days past due. Therefore, every hospital has an automatic 30-day extension. The intermediary can apply verbal pressure within the 30 days if an extension was not approved, but cannot do anything else.

The hospital statement of reimbursable cost (Medicare cost report) is the most important document filed annually by most hospitals. This report is both challenging and rewarding. It does not utilize double-entry principles of accounting; therefore, an error in transposition or in a mathematical calculation will not automatically reveal itself. For many of the schedules, there is nothing to tie to. In addition, it must be remembered that the regulations are not simple, direct, and explicit. Therefore, it is important to have the cost report completed, or at least reviewed, by a person who is familiar with cost reporting principles. Computer systems can eliminate most of the mathematical errors, but they do very little to maximize reimbursement.

The Medicare maximization review should not be performed by the same person every year. Medicare maximization requires creative thinking, and fresh ideas seldom evolve from reviewing data with which we are already familiar.

Provider Reimbursement Review Board

The use of intermediaries between the government and the provider of medical care started as an experiment between the government and the private sector. By the early 1970s, however, it became apparent that equivocal interpretations of the regulations were counterproductive to the needs of both the hospitals and the intermediaries.

The Provider Reimbursement Review Board (PRRB) was established on December 18, 1974. The PRRB is bound by the regulations but is not bound by intermediary letters or by any of the health insurance manuals. They do, however, give great weight to the manuals.

To be considered by the PRRB, there must be at least $10,000 of reimbursement in question; on a group appeal there must be $50,000 of reimbursement in question. If there is not enough money being questioned to bring the matter before the PRRB, the hospital has two options: It can appeal the matter through the Blue Cross appeal process, or the amount in question can be artificially inflated. Artificially inflating the amount in question is accomplished by adding items to the appeal that you would not otherwise question.

Decisions of the PRRB are not precedent setting. This means that a ruling on any one year in the cost report does not affect other years. Rulings also do not affect other providers. Therefore, a separate and distinct appeal must be made to the PRRB each year by each provider even if the controversy is the same. The PRRB will be discussed at length in later chapters.

Frame of Reference

It is important to view reimbursement as a "no-limits" report. Many hospitals complain bitterly about cost report restrictions, yet they are entitled to hundreds of thousands of dollars in additional reimbursement. They do not perform the maximization techniques that are available. Some hospitals believe that, if they are paying an outside firm to complete the cost reports, they must be getting all the reimbursement possible. However, outside firms often prepare safe reports that do not maximize reimbursement.

An example from a state with a Blue Cross cost report for hospitals illustrates these self-imposed cost report limitations. Over the years in this state, the Blue Cross plan has on several occasions changed the forms for filing its cost reports. Each time the forms were changed, they became more restrictive. The original contract between Blue Cross and the hospitals has never been changed. Yet, reportedly, not a single hospital in the state has ever questioned the authority of the plan to make changes in the cost reporting forms. A careful review of the contract would reveal that very little of the present cost report schedules are authorized in the contract. Thus, the hospitals are complaining about a set of forms that they are not required to use.

In several states, the Blue Cross contract stipulates that allowable costs will be determined according to generally accepted accounting principles. When Medicare changes the manner in which costs are determined, the Blue Cross cost reporting forms are changed accordingly. The hospitals in these states are losing millions of dollars in reimbursement because they are beguiled by cost reporting forms that are being changed according to Medicare principles of reimbursement rather than generally accepted accounting principles, as called for in the contract.

Later, in the chapter on appeals and controversies, we make it clear that cost reimbursement is more of a frame of reference than a knowledge of rules and regulations. Hospitals, nursing homes, and other providers throughout the country are losing millions of dollars in allowable reimbursement because they believe nothing can be done. As we will show, however, there is a lot that can be done. New financial regulations in the future may make parts of this book irrelevant; however, the general principles discussed should remain relevant for many years.

PROSPECTIVE PAYMENT SYSTEMS

There is a growing awareness of the fact that both the government and the health care industry would benefit from prospective, rather than retrospective, reimbursement. Prospective reimbursement will allow the government to predict its budget and to anticipate with certainty the outcome of proposed new regulations. The present retrospective reimbursement system has become too complex to estimate the savings of proposed new regulations with any degree of accuracy. Also, it does not give the government the desired control over health care costs.

Prospective payment will be an advantage to health care providers because it will allow them to know in advance how much the government will pay for Medicare and Medicaid patients. This will allow the hospitals and other entities to make appropriate financial decisions. Sometimes the appropriate decision will be to lower the quality of care being given.

The preliminary regulations exclude capital costs, education costs, and outpatient costs from prospective payment. This will make capital decisions that reduce operating costs prudent decisions, even if the reductions are relatively small and the required capital costs are relatively large. The health care industry will become less labor intensive. There will also be a trend toward more outpatient procedures. If the currently proposed regulations are enacted, providers should start to shift costs from inpatient to outpatient areas in order to maximize reimbursement.

Payment Systems by Diagnosis

Commercial insurance companies and the preferred provider organizations are studying systems of prospective payment by diagnosis as a way to reimburse hospitals. Hospitals must carefully negotiate any prospective payment system with nongovernment payers. The government will continue to pay less than cost for Medicare and Medicaid patients, thus requiring hospitals to shift costs to other payers. Any prospective payment with commercial insurance payers must allow the hospital to collect more than reasonable cost, plus a reasonable markup. If a hospital received less than cost for government patients and received only reasonable costs for other patients, there would be no opportunity to break even. Bankruptcy would be inevitable. The only question would be how long the institution could survive with an eroding financial base.

Prospective payment by diagnosis will place increased importance on peer review, discharge planning, and medical records. Computer systems for peer review and discharge planning are being developed to identify physicians who order excessive ancillary tests or who have excessive inpatient days. Medical records will be required to place as high a diagnosis as possible on patient stays, as well as to identify complications that require patient stays beyond average length. The preliminary regulations provide for additional payment for ''outlier'' cases. The only department that can identify outlier cases and provide the documentation for obtaining additional reimbursement is medical records. Eventually this process will be computerized in most hospitals.

Table 1–1 shows a discharge patient analysis from a computer program based on prospective payment by diagnosis. This program also produces a hospital discharge abstract for every patient, a diagnosis delinquency

Table 1–1 Discharge Patient Analysis

ICD Number		Physician	Patient		Length of Stay				Charges			Reference
Primary	Secondary	Name	No.	Name	Act.	Std.	Var.	Act.	Std.	Var.		Reference
410.9	410.4	Smith	1234	Jones	21	23	(2)	8912	10,012	(1100)		18
386.3	—	Jones	1235	Smith	6	4	2	1200	1100	1000		23
389.9	386.3	Taylor	1236	Graham	7	7	0	1350	1300	50		33
414.0	—	Carpenter	1237	Lee	2	3	1	680	720	(40)		12

report with total dollars (per case as well as per physician), and a detailed patient analysis by diagnosis. The information necessary to update the daily reports is keyed into a computer terminal located in medical records at the hospital that uses the system.

The Table 1–1 analysis shows the primary ICD diagnosis and, if applicable, the secondary diagnosis. It identifies the doctor, the admission number, and the patient. Then, for every discharge, the analysis shows the actual length of stay, the standard length of stay, and the variance. The actual gross charges, the standard gross charges, and the charge variance for the diagnosis are shown. The reference column cites the detailed report on the admission summarized on that particular line.

Computer reports like that in Table 1–1 can be summarized by physician or by diagnosis so that the hospital can identify the profitability of both the physicians and the diagnoses. The reports can be shown by financial class or in total. They can also be programmed to show only exceptions by length of stay or by gross charges, according to predetermined variance limits set by the hospital.

Prospective payment will dramatically change health care delivery. The annual physician credentialing process will be used to censor physicians who are not profitable, and rewards for efficient case managing will be given. In many hospitals, medical records and discharge planning will report to the chief financial officer. The budget process will become more sophisticated, and all hospital departments will be affected.

All these financial requirements will take a minimum of two years to perfect. Hospitals that do not start early will not survive. However, the hospitals that do survive will be better managed and financially stronger than the hospitals of the past.

Case Mix Management

In order to manage by case mix, hospitals must have a five-part data base, consisting of:

1. historical case mix
2. current case mix
3. standard costs per diagnosis
4. standard length of stay per diagnosis
5. physician reports by diagnosis, covering length of stay, ancillaries ordered, and payer mix.

The first action requirement is to assemble a task force composed of finance, medical records, medical staff, admitting, and nursing. The task force leader should be given specific objectives and due dates for their completion. All information by diagnosis must be centralized in a common data base. This includes information presently available in medical records and billing. Unless the information from these two areas is centralized, the hospital cannot perform effective case mix management.

There is a need for financial clinical meetings to exchange information. The financial people must understand the concerns of the medical staff, and the medical staff should be made aware of the financial requirements imposed by third party payers. Through these meetings, standards for length of stay and for ancillaries ordered by diagnosis can be developed. The physicians can also suggest capital equipment that will reduce operating costs.

Hospitals that do not have adequate data processing capabilities will find management by case mix extremely difficult because the volume of data is so great. Hospitals should reevaluate their data processing needs and their present data processing activities. Rather than purchase new equipment with more capacity, it may be more prudent to eliminate some of the present reports and replace them with information needed to manage by case mix. As the information needs change, many of the reports designed to make decisions or to manage under the old rules are no longer relevant. Thus the task force should reevaluate the present reports. Most hospitals should not need additional data processing capabilities to manage case mix reimbursement and prospective payment systems.

Cost containment under case mix management should be carefully planned so that the areas that contribute to the hospital receive the most budget funds and budget cuts are made in the areas that support nonprofitable diagnoses. Many hospitals will have to cut expenses in all departments to remain financially solvent.

NOTES

1. Sec. 102(a) of SS Amendments of 1965 (P.L. 89-97).

Chapter 2

Overview of Principles

ANNUAL COST INCREASES

The Container of Costs

Assume that all costs necessary to staff and operate the hospital are in a container like that shown in Figure 2–1. Each year two additional kinds of cost are added to the container.

Historically, two thirds of the cost increases each year have been normal inflationary increases. These include salary increases, increases for fringe benefits, price increases for suppliers, increases in utility costs, increases in services, replacement of fixed assets at inflated prices and other increases. These increases would be present in any industry; they are not unique to hospitals.

Approximately one third of the increases in hospital costs each year have historically been due to new and better services. These are due to greater patient acuity because of a shorter average length of stay, increases in the number of tests performed per patient day, new drugs, technology that is new to the hospital, and average salary rate increases resulting from the need for higher skill levels.

Cost increases resulting from new and better services are related to patient acuity. Average patient acuity is increased when old procedures are transferred from the hospital setting to an outpatient setting, such as a physician's office. It is also increased when the hospital dispenses drugs that were not available a few years ago or performs diagnostic tests that the hospital could not perform in the past. Every hospital has more sophisticated diagnostic and treatment equipment than it did a few years ago. To measure patient acuity, we must evaluate each hospital individually. It makes no difference how long a procedure or a piece of equipment has been in use by other hospitals in the area. The first year the procedure or

Figure 2–1 Container of Costs Needed To Run a Hospital

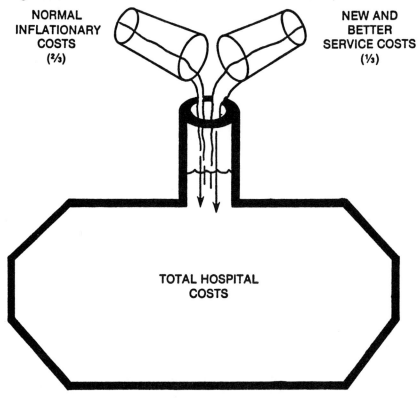

NORMAL
INFLATIONARY
COSTS
(⅔)

NEW AND
BETTER
SERVICE COSTS
(⅓)

TOTAL HOSPITAL
COSTS

Source: Reprinted from *Basic Hospital Financial Management* by D.F. Beck, with permission of Aspen Systems Corp., Rockville, Md., © 1980.

the equipment is available in a particular hospital, it increases the technology available to serve that hospital's patients. Therefore, the cost to provide that service is due to new and better ways of operating the hospital. In the Figure 2–1 example, if costs were to increase by $15 per patient day, we would know that approximately $10 of that was due to inflation and approximately $5 was due to providing new and better services.

Distribution of Cost Increases

As we pour additional costs into the container each year, they must be absorbed somewhere. Let us assume that our container has four standpipes to absorb new costs, as in Figure 2–2. There are standpipes for Medicare,

Figure 2–2 Container of Hospital Costs with Cost-Absorbing Standpipes

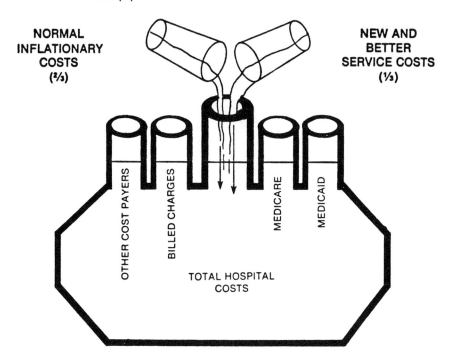

NORMAL
INFLATIONARY
COSTS
(⅔)

NEW AND
BETTER
SERVICE COSTS
(⅓)

OTHER COST PAYERS

BILLED CHARGES

MEDICARE

MEDICAID

TOTAL HOSPITAL
COSTS

Source: Reprinted from *Basic Hospital Financial Management* by D.F. Beck, with permission of Aspen Systems Corp., Rockville, Md., © 1980.

Medicaid, billed charges payers, and other cost payers. The latter are non-Medicare and non-Medicaid payers who reimburse the hospital on a basis other than billed charges. This includes Blue Cross in about half of the states. It also includes payers of costs covered by special agreement with social agencies, health maintenance organizations, and government programs that pay on a per diem regardless of how that per diem is computed; by contracts with other providers; and by other programs that do not pay billed charges.

Billed charges refer to patient revenue that is covered by payers whose payments are based on the hospital's actual billed charges. Such payers include most commercial insurance companies, patients who pay all or part of their charges, and some social agencies. Billed charges do not include amounts for bad debts, charity, contractual allowances, and other deductions from revenue. The hospital cannot pass cost increases on to patients who do not pay. The Medicare and Medicaid standpipes cover only the portion of the patient's charges that are covered by the applicable program. Patient coinsurance and deductible amounts are included in the standpipe for billed charges.

Cost-Based Third Party Payers

As we add costs to our container each year, we would expect each standpipe to absorb its share of the costs. However, that is not what happens. Medicare, Medicaid, and other cost payers control the amount of cost increases they will absorb. Historically, cost payers have absorbed significantly less than their share of additional costs each year. This is illustrated by the Figure 2–3 container, which has stopcocks in the standpipes for cost payers.

Figure 2–3 Container of Hospital Costs with Stopcock Constraints on Cost-Absorbing Standpipes

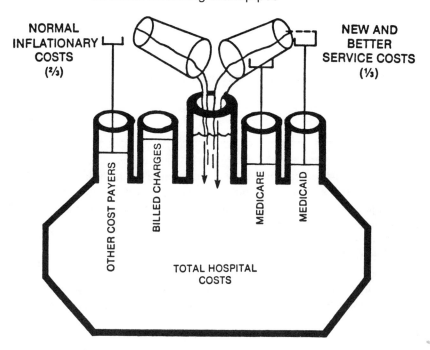

Source: Reprinted from *Basic Hospital Financial Management* by D.F. Beck, with permission of Aspen Systems Corp., Rockville, Md., © 1980.

The stopcocks are the cost reports. Cost payers can push down on their stopcock, forcing more costs into the other standpipes; they can freeze the stopcock at the current level; or they can release the stopcock to absorb a portion of the cost increases. In the Figure 2–3 container, there is a dotted line connecting the Medicare and Medicaid standpipes. This is because the principles of reimbursement for the two programs are similar. Medicaid reimbursement normally is determined by Medicare reimbursement. The hospital completes its Medicare cost report first. The Medicaid report either uses the same forms or refers to lines on one of the Medicare forms.

In the past, Medicare and Medicaid have absorbed significantly less than their share of the additional costs each year. Blue Cross and other cost payers have generally absorbed their share of cost increases, but no more. Billed charge payers thus have had to absorb their share of the costs as well as cost increases attributable to Medicare, Medicaid, and other government patients. It is important to remember that as long as a payer is on a cost contract, the stopcock will not be raised to absorb all increases in hospital charges. Cost payers ignore prices. It should also be remembered that the majority of cost payers are government payers, and the hospital will thus receive less than cost for their patients.

It should be obvious from the above discussion that hospitals have been forced to raise prices to billed charge payers by an amount that passes on to these payers a disproportionate share of health care costs. This is commonly called cost shifting. As the hospitals receive less than cost from government patients, they attempt to shift more costs to billed charge patients.

It is important to note that in those states in which Blue Cross reimburses on a cost contract, Blue Cross will have a distinct and measurable price advantage over other health insurance companies. In those states in which Blue Cross reimburses on billed charges, it still has a small price advantage over other insurance companies. In these states, Blue Cross usually pays a discounted amount or has other advantages.

THE COST DILEMMA

It should be clear from the above discussion that hospital price increases generally affect only that class of patients who pay billed charges. The majority of hospital patients ignore the prices. The following formula can be used to estimate the net effect of a price increase:

$$PI = 100 - (CR + BD + CC)$$

where: PI = Percentage increase from price increase
        CR = Percentage of revenue that is cost reimbursed
        BD = Percentage of revenue that is bad debts
        CC = Percentage of revenue that is charity care

Assume that a hospital is 60 percent cost reimbursed, has 6-percent bad debts, and has 4-percent chare. Using our formula, the percentage increase from price incre   100 − (60 + 6 + 4) = 30 percent.

In this example, 70   ital's patients ignore prices, and 30 percent of the p   . If this hospital raises prices by $1 million, it   and deductions from gross revenue will i   1 million from the price increases, t   ces by over $3.3 million.

If a ho   ursed spends an additional $1 million, it   al reimbursement simply because the money w   e hospital that is 60-percent cost reimbursed redu   illion, $600,000 of this saving accrues to the cost payers a   al realizes only $400,000.

Thus, the patient m   determines the financial viability of a hospital. A high percentage cost payer patients leaves fewer patients upon whom the hospital can transfer the loss realized on government patients. With a small percentage of cost payer patients, there is a higher portion of patients to whom the hospital can transfer its costs.

The Figure 2–4 container illustrates the cost dilemma faced by American hospitals and other providers. Here, Medicare and Medicaid pay less than cost; other cost payers pay more than Medicare and Medicaid but not full billed charges; and billed charge payers pay significantly more than their share of costs.

The billed charge payers are at the economic spillover point. The spillover point is that economic point at which patients, insurance companies, social agencies, and others in the billed charge category either cannot or will not pay the hospital's published charges within a reasonable time period. The hospitals continue to raise prices, and state insurance commissioners refuse to grant commercial insurance companies the full requested rate increases. The commercial insurance companies have, therefore, extended their payment time lag.

There are several strategies a hospital with a high percentage of cost reimbursement can follow. The first strategy is to reduce the amount of cost increases each year. If a hospital reduces the amount spent for new and better services more than other hospitals in its service area, it will soon fall behind. A hospital with outdated equipment and technology will soon lose the loyalty of its medical staff and, therefore, its revenue. A

Figure 2–4 Container of Hospital Costs with Billed-Charge Payers at the Economic Spillover Point

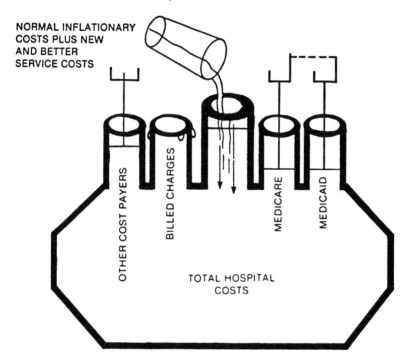

Source: Reprinted from *Basic Hospital Financial Management* by D.F. Beck, with permission of Aspen Systems Corp., Rockville, Md., © 1980.

hospital must be very cautious in determining the amount of reductions in new and better service costs. A second strategy is to attempt to make reductions in the amount of normal price increases; but a hospital has only limited control over these increases, and the gains will be small. A third strategy is to reduce the amount of costs in the container. A word of caution, however: Over time, significant reductions in existing costs will reduce the service level and reverse gains made in prior years. This will cause the hospital to lose the loyalty of its medical staff.

The hospitals and other health care providers continue to receive reduced revenues from Medicare, Medicaid, and other cost payers to cover rising costs. It is becoming more difficult to transfer these costs to billed charge payers because the latter are at an economic spillover point. If a hospital attempts to reduce spending, there is the risk of losing the loyalty of the medical staff and, therefore, its revenue.

To remain financially viable, hospitals must become more aggressive with cost reimbursement, with third party payers, and with corporate restructuring. We hope this book will help in these areas.

DEFINITION OF MEDICARE COSTS

In this section, our discussion of the principles relating to Medicare applies as well to Medicaid (Title 19), crippled children (Title 5), and other cost payers. Medicare cost reports are uniform throughout the United States and are generally the starting point for other cost reports. Other cost systems are either modeled after the Medicare cost reimbursement system or have many principles in common with Medicare reimbursement. (Appendix A contains general instructions for the hospital Medicare cost report that were applicable at this writing. These instructions should be reviewed in conjunction with this chapter to gain a better understanding of the cost report process.)

Total Costs

The Medicare reimbursement system is outlined in Table 2–1. The first component is total costs as defined by generally accepted accounting principles (GAAP). The last component is true reimbursement, which is what the government ultimately pays. The components between these two give the government an opportunity to pay less than cost.

Table 2–1 Third Party Payer, Cost Reimbursement System

Total costs	$XXXX
Less defined-away costs	XX
Allowable costs	XXXX
Less offsets & adjustments	XX
Costs to be apportioned	XXXX
Less apportioned-away costs	XX
Recognized patient costs	XXXX
Less nonprogram costs	XXX
Allowable costs	XXX
Less limits & ceilings	X
Recognized program costs	XXX
Plus return on equity	XX
Reimbursed costs	XXX
Less inflation shrinkage	XX
True reimbursement	$ XXX

Although total costs are defined in the hospital's accounting system, this is not the starting point for Medicare. All hospitals have some costs that can be added for cost report purposes. The most significant costs to be added are those from a related organization. Anything that a related organization does for the hospital can be calculated and added for Medicare purposes. This includes, but is not limited to, snow removal, interest expense, administrative overhead, and depreciation on donated assets. This rule applies to city, county, and state hospitals, as well as those owned by religious orders and chains.

Hospitals can also impute a cost for certain volunteer services. Depreciation is allowed on donated assets, even though there was no cash outlay. Specific techniques on how to add to total costs will be covered in subsequent chapters. For now it is important to remember only that all providers normally have some costs that can be added to costs as determined by GAAP.

Defined-Away Costs

It has been estimated that the Medicare and Medicaid programs reimburse hospitals for about 80 percent of actual costs. This means that whenever the hospital admits a Medicare or Medicaid patient, it is known that the hospital will experience a loss. The first deduction from costs in Table 2–1 is that for defined-away costs. Examples of such costs are those for patient telephones, patient television, professional office buildings, coffee shops, bad debts, discounts, and physician recruitment fees.

For cost report purposes, the hospital simply does not include the cost of items that have been defined away for Medicare purposes, though they are still recognized as costs according to GAAP. In subsequent chapters we examine specific ways in which defined-away costs can be minimized.

Offsets and Adjustments

After the adjustment for defined-away costs, the Table 2–1 cost report system shows allowable costs. The regulations require an offset or adjustment to allowable costs for almost all nonpatient sources of income. These offsets are made on Medicare Schedule A–8. At the time of this writing, the Schedule A–8 adjustments represent the area where American hospitals and other providers are losing the largest amount of potential additional reimbursement.

Examples of required offsets and adjustments include those for silver recovery, telephone rebates, cafeteria income, medical records abstracts, vending machine income, cot rentals, and shared service income. The regulations require the hospital to offset cash received for each category of costs if the costs can be determined. Almost without exception, the costs are significantly less than the cash received. The regulations state that the hospital can make a profit on these sources of income and keep the profit, if it can be determined. Many hospitals offset cash received because it is a readily available figure.

Techniques to minimize offsets and adjustments and thereby maximize program reimbursement are covered in Chapter 4. These techniques are simple, straightforward, and normally result in significant additional reimbursement.

Apportioned-Away Costs

After offsets and adjustments, the cost report process in Table 2–1 moves to costs to be apportioned. Medicare, Medicaid, and other payers pay only for services performed by revenue-producing departments. To be paid for housekeeping, maintenance, dietary services, administration, and the services of other nonrevenue-producing departments, the costs of these departments must be allocated to the revenue-producing departments. This is accomplished on a schedule called the Medicare stepdown. Statistics, cost studies, and other bases are used in the process.

In selecting, as well as in developing statistics, the hospital should attempt to allocate as much cost as possible to the high-cost-reimbursed departments. If the hospital is at one of the cost-reimbursement limits, the costs should be allocated away from the department at the reimbursement limit and into departments that do not have such limits. Other ways to minimize the amount of costs apportioned away include direct costing, timing the preparation of the required studies, and corporate reorganizations. These and other techniques are discussed in Chapter 5.

Nonprogram Costs

From recognized patient costs in Table 2–1, the reimbursement system subtracts nonprogram costs. This is accomplished on schedule C through a formula called the charge converter:

$$\frac{\text{Program revenue}}{\text{Total gross revenue}} \times \begin{array}{c}\text{Allowable}\\\text{costs}\end{array} = \begin{array}{c}\text{What the}\\\text{hospital receives}\end{array}$$

This formula is applied for every ancillary department. It should be remembered that allowable costs are significantly less than the real costs as defined by GAAP.

As discussed in Chapter 6, hospitals and other health care providers can maximize reimbursement through a comprehensive pricing strategy. After the overall hospital price increase has been determined, pricing strategy is used to determine which departments receive a greater percentage markup than others. The logic in pricing strategy is the reverse of that in the techniques used in placing expenses. The hospital attempts to put the largest price increases in those departments that have the greatest propensity to be billed-charge reimbursed. Conversely, the hospital attempts to place the largest amount of costs in those departments that have the greatest propensity to be cost reimbursed.

Once departmental price increases have been determined, the hospital reviews individual procedures within each department. Raising the prices of some procedures more than others within a department can result in a greater net profit.

Limits and Ceilings

After nonprogram costs have been culled out, the cost reimbursement system of Table 2–1 defines allowable costs as determined by the Health Care Financing Administration. At this writing, there are reimbursement limits on routine care and two limits on cost per case, pharmacy drugs, respiratory therapy if under contract, physical therapy if under contract, and other therapy services. The two limits on costs per case were enacted as part of the Tax Equity and Fiscal Responsibility Act (TEFRA) of 1982. One was a target rate limit that compared costs per case with national costs per case, and the other compared costs per case with the hospital's actual costs per case. Other ceilings have been proposed and are being studied.

Limits and ceilings stipulate arbitrary amounts that limit reimbursement. Once a ceiling or limit is reached, no additional reimbursement can be obtained, regardless of the propriety of the expenditure. Most of these limits and ceilings were established as budget-balancing measures. Additional limits and ceilings are almost certain in the future because they are relatively easy to implement and monitor. In addition, they can save billions of dollars for the government.

When a hospital reaches one of these limits, cost shifting should be attempted. By shifting costs out of the area where they cannot be reimbursed and into an area where there is no limit, reimbursement can be maximized. Another tactic is to request an exception from the limit or ceiling. Exemptions are difficult to obtain but are possible with enough documentation. These techniques are explained more fully in subsequent chapters.

Return on Equity

After adjusting for limits and ceilings, the cost process moves to recognized program costs. These are allowable reimbursements according to the current regulations. Return on equity is allowed as an addition to recognized program costs on cost reports for proprietary and other for-profit providers. At this writing, nonprofit providers do not receive a return on equity. Many knowledgeable observers feel that tax-exempt hospitals will never receive a return on equity because of the policies of the Internal Revenue Service (IRS) regarding tax-exempt institutions. Others believe that tax-exempt hospitals may some day be allowed to add a return-on-equity calculation to their allowable costs.

Return on equity is based upon the amount of money invested in fixed assets, plus the amount of net working capital. This amount is multiplied by the average interest paid in the past year on government securities. Because a return on equity is paid on fixed assets, there is an incentive to capitalize assets that would normally be expensed in a tax-exempt institution. Under the current law, the for-profit hospital receives significant tax advantages, including investment credits and an accelerated depreciation write-off for tax purposes. For-profit hospital accounting policies normally capitalize more assets than the accounting policies of tax-exempt hospitals.

Another tactic successfully used by some for-profit hospitals to increase their return on equity is to inflate working capital artificially. This can be accomplished by increasing current assets or by decreasing current liabilities. Techniques to accomplish this are discussed in detail in subsequent chapters.

In tax-exempt institutions, recognized program costs are identical to reimbursed costs. In for-profit institutions, return on equity is added to recognized program costs to arrive at reimbursed costs.

Inflation Shrinkage

Inflation shrinkage refers to attempts in the Medicare and Medicaid programs to delay payment as long as possible. With inflation, the funds are then repaid in cheaper dollars, or dollars that have less purchasing power. For example, if someone owes you $100 today and that person withholds payment for a year in which there is ten-percent inflation, you will be repaid in funds that have an equivalent purchasing power of $90. In inflationary times, it is an advantage to delay payment as long as possible. The advantage is in direct proportion to the rate of inflation.

Hospitals are reimbursed for Medicare according to a negotiated interim rate. It is important to remember that this interim rate is negotiated and not set by the intermediary. To understand how the interim rate works, let us examine the IRS tax-withholding system. Throughout the year, employees have an estimated amount withheld from their paycheck for federal income taxes. At year end, the employees complete a tax return to determine their true tax liability. The calculated tax liability is compared to the amount withheld as an estimate throughout the year. Upon filing their tax returns, the employees either ask for a refund or, if the withheld amount is less than their tax liability, attach a check to their return.

The interim rate for Medicare works exactly the same way. An estimate is made of the amount of reimbursement, and the hospital's interim rate is determined. If the interim rate is 80 percent, then for every $100,000 in billed charges the hospital will be given $80,000. At year end, a Medicare cost report is completed to determine the true reimbursement. The reimbursement is compared to the amount collected at the interim rate, and the hospital either requests a refund or attaches a check to its cost report when it is filed.

It is not a coincidence that many elements of the Medicare program resemble rules and procedures used by the IRS. At the inception of the Medicare program in 1965, there was no Medicare Bureau to write rules for this new government program. Several agents were transferred from the IRS to accomplish this. They brought with them their IRS indoctrination, knowledge of practice, and systems.

It is to the government's advantage to make the interim rate as low as possible so that the hospital always has a refund due at year end. It normally takes at least 3 months after year end to file the cost reports and another 1 or 2 months to complete the desk audit of the cost reports and obtain an interim settlement. Therefore, funds are withheld not only for the 12 months of the fiscal year but up to 5 months beyond the fiscal year end. It is to the hospital's advantage to owe money at the time the cost reports are filed.

A technique that delays payment to the hospital is to perform an interim rate review based on the first quarter of operations. This is the least expensive quarter because it does not contain any part of the last nine months' inflation. Often, and especially if the fiscal year ends on December 31, the first quarter is also the most efficient quarter in terms of productivity. By using this "cheap" quarter to project the rest of the year, the hospital's interim rate is lowered to an inappropriate amount, and a significant refund is due at year end.

Another area in which inflation shrinkage works against the hospitals is in disputes between the intermediary and the provider. Money is withheld from current billings to the hospital as if the intermediary will win all disputes. If the matter is finally decided by the courts, it may take as long as four or five years. If the hospital then wins the dispute, it is paid the original amount, but without interest or an adjustment for inflation. Techniques to reduce inflation shrinkage are examined in subsequent chapters.

COST REIMBURSEMENT STRATEGIES

The cost reimbursement system has become more and more unfavorable to hospitals and other providers in the years since its inception in 1967. Most of the regulations that represent a departure from GAAP were initiated by the Medicare Bureau in order to balance its budget. There simply has not been enough funds to pay for all of the health care promised in the Medicare, Medicaid, and the other government programs.

In future years, the system will become even more restrictive as the government continues to attempt to reduce federal deficits. Hospitals will continue to transfer a disproportionate share of their cost increases on to commercial insurance companies and others that pay billed charges. As the difference between total cost and true reimbursement grows, this tactic will become more difficult, especially for those institutions with a relatively large percentage of cost reimbursed patients. It is, therefore, imperative that hospitals carefully examine each step in the cost reimbursement system to determine strategies that can be used to maximize reimbursement.

One of the strategies that is being used increasingly is corporate reorganization. Institutions are identifying those areas that restrict cost reimbursement the most and are transferring functions from these areas to a foundation or other corporate entity. For example, where the cost of a professional office building has been defined away from Medicare, it is to a hospital's advantage to give the building to another corporate entity. If a separate corporation owns the building, there are no costs to be offset or disallowed on the hospital's cost report. If a source of revenue results in an offset or adjustment on Schedule A–8 of the cost report, that source is transferred to another corporate entity. Then there is nothing to be offset.

The trend toward corporate reorganizations and hospital takeovers by large chains has been due to a large extent to current reimbursement regulations. (Corporate reorganizations are discussed in detail in Chapter 9.)

If a hospital does not become more aggressive in its cost reports, move toward corporate reorganization, do market analysis, and adopt a marketing strategy to determine its patient mix, it will most likely not survive. Some that do not survive will go bankrupt; others will be purchased or leased by large chains.

BLUE CROSS COST REPORTS

In approximately half of the states, Blue Cross reimburses hospitals according to a cost report. In the other half, Blue Cross reimburses billed charges but, because it is such a large payer, exerts much of the influence it would have with a cost report. Even in those states where Blue Cross is not on a cost report, it customarily pays less than full billed charges. The present section discusses primarily Blue Cross cost reports, but the principles are applicable to all contracts with Blue Cross.

An Overview

Blue Cross plans usually have a contract with the hospital. Many years ago, there was no reason to study the terms of the contract carefully because Blue Cross plans were run or controlled by the hospitals. The goals of both parties were the same. Two things have occurred to change this relationship. The first has been the role of Blue Cross plans as intermediaries for Medicare. The second has been the financial hardship imposed on Blue Cross and other commercial insurance companies because of cost shifting.

Many Blue Cross contracts stipulate that costs will be determined according to GAAP. It is important to remember that GAAP are promulgated by the American Institute of CPAs or the Financial Accounting Standards Board; they are not promulgated by the Medicare Bureau. As Medicare principles increasingly restrict payments to hospitals, there is a tendency on the part of Blue Cross plans to adopt the same restrictive principles in their reimbursement to hospitals for Blue Cross patients. Blue Cross officials know Medicare principles well because they have implemented them as Medicare intermediaries. These officials regard those principles as logical. Add to this the fact that Blue Cross plans are suffering financially because of cost shifting.

The hospitals over the years have grown to trust Blue Cross and to accept the Medicare principles of reimbursement. The whole process seems logical and predictable. By accepting this situation, many hospitals are losing hundreds of thousands of dollars in allowable reimbursement on their Blue Cross cost reports. In fact, it is important for hospitals to forget Medicare principles when completing the Blue Cross cost report. Those cost reports should be completed using the language of the contract.

Application of Principles

Many Blue Cross plans have amended their cost reports several times in recent years. Often these amendments have been made without a change in the contract. New schedules, new instructions, and new principles are sent to all applicable hospitals with a cover letter stating that the new forms should be used for the next cost report. The new forms are normally less favorable to the hospital, yet many hospitals have blindly followed the instructions and have used the new forms.

A common example of this is in the offsets and adjustments that are required by Medicare on Schedule A–8. These are not based on GAAP. Unless the Blue Cross contract specifically requires that these offsets and adjustments be made, a hospital should not complete any schedule on the Blue Cross cost report that requires that they be made. Another example is a part of the Blue Cross cost report that eliminates some of the Medicare defined-away costs. Costs that are not recognized as patient-care-related for Medicare should be included on the Blue Cross report unless the Blue Cross contract specifically excludes them. Other examples of Medicare principles that may be assumed to pertain to the Blue Cross cost report include the grossing up of discounted prices to special patients such as referred laboratory patients, a disallowance of bad debts and charity, and the setting of certain limits and ceilings.

Obviously, one cannot address specifically all of the Blue Cross cost reports in America in one book. In general, however, it can be concluded that a hospital should examine the current Blue Cross cost report carefully and compare each segment or line with the language in the Blue Cross contract. This review should be performed either by an aggressive, competent financial analyst or by someone totally unfamiliar with Medicare principles. Anything on the Blue Cross cost report that is not required by contract can be challenged to effect additional reimbursement.

Disputes about the Blue Cross contract can be taken to local courts. Such disputes are settled according to contract law, which is not as unfavorable to hospitals as Medicare principles. Hospitals should be aware, however, that, if an adverse schedule or other part of the Blue Cross cost report has been completed for several years even though it is not required by contract, a precedent has been set. The court may rule that the point being contested is not clear and, therefore, rule in favor of Blue Cross because of precedent. For this reason, hospitals should study changes in their cost reports very carefully in order to prevent the establishment of a new unnecessary precedent that reduces reimbursement.

Often Blue Cross will offer a hospital a new Blue Cross contract, stating that there are shortcomings in the old contract. This happens with Blue Cross plans that reimburse on a form of billed charges as well as with plans that reimburse on a cost contract. It is important to review every contract change to determine if it is in the best interest of the hospital to sign. Many hospitals have signed new contracts or addenda to contracts that have cost them literally millions of dollars in additional reimbursement from Blue Cross over a period of years. Thus, it is recommended that all Blue Cross contract changes be reviewed by a reimbursement expert as well as by an attorney.

The important points to remember about reimbursement are that it is not always logical or just and that many reimbursement limits are self-imposed. The hospital that is not creative and aggressive in its reimbursement posture probably will not survive in today's economic climate.

Chapter 3

Appeals and Controversies

THE MEDICARE HIERARCHY

The Statutory and Regulatory Framework

Figure 3–1 illustrates the Medicare hierarchy. It begins with the constitution, the law of the land by which we are all bound. Under the constitution is the Congress, which passed the original statute that created Medicare: Public Law 92–603, titled the Social Security Amendments of 1965. Since this act was signed into law on October 20, 1965, the amendments have been changed every year. In some years the changes were only minor; in other years, they produced sweeping changes in the Medicare system. In any event, we are all bound by the statutes passed under the constitution by Congress.

In the social security statutes, Congress gave the secretary of HHS the authority to interpret the intent of Congress and to issue regulations governing the Medicare program. Hospitals, nursing homes, and other providers are bound by the secretary's regulations, as perfected. They are not bound by regulations that have not been perfected. To perfect a regulation, the secretary must publish the regulation in the Federal Register, allow time for comment, and make the regulations final. This protects the providers from sudden or retroactive regulations.

As shown in Figure 3–1, the courts and the providers are not bound by anything beyond the HHS regulations. The charter of the PRRB states that it is not bound by the health insurance manuals, intermediary letters, or other rules. However, in the majority of hearings, the PRRB acts as if it were bound by the manuals and rulings. Therefore, the PRRB is placed below the courts and providers with the intermediaries.

Below the secretary of HHS is the Health Care Financing Administration (HCFA). HCFA issues rulings, manuals, policy statements, general

Figure 3–1 The Medicare Hierarchy

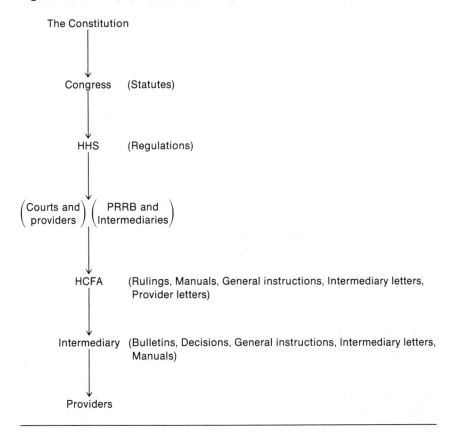

instructions, and intermediary letters. By contract, the intermediaries are bound by all HCFA rules and regulations. However, hospitals are not bound by them. The best-known manuals are Health Insurance Manual 10 (HIM–10), which explains coverage and billing instructions, and Health Insurance Manual 15 (HIM–15), which explains the cost report process. HIM–10 is the billing manual, and HIM–15 is the provider manual. But, as noted, the providers are not bound by these; their contract is with the secretary of HHS.

Below the HCFA in Figure 3–1 is the intermediary. The main intermediary is Blue Cross America (BCA) in Chicago. BCA has subcontracted their intermediary function to local Blue Cross plans throughout the nation. Over the years, BCA has issued bulletins, decisions, general instructions, intermediary letters, and manuals. By contract, the local intermediaries are bound by these. The hospitals and other providers are not bound by them.

It should be clear by now that the intermediary is bound by contract to follow an impressive amount of regulations and other rules that the provider is not bound by. The intermediary rules are very different from those of the providers. Therefore, if a hospital has a question on interpretation of the regulations, it is not appropriate to ask the intermediary. The intermediary can only interpret through the manuals, rulings, policies, and other information that bind it.

It should be noted, however, that the vast majority of the information in HIM–10, HIM–15, intermediary letters, and other similar sources serves to clarify the secretary's regulations. For this purpose, this material is very useful. Every hospital, nursing home, and other provider should have updated copies of the HCFA manuals. The manuals as well as revisions should be provided free by the intermediary. Yet, although most of this material serves to clarify, hospitals and other providers must keep in mind that they are not bound by it. There can and should be numerous areas of disagreement.

Choice of Intermediary

Hospitals and other providers can choose their intermediary. Historically, most hospitals have chosen Blue Cross as their Part-A intermediary. However, from a theoretical point of view, Blue Cross was the worst choice. As indicated in Figure 3–1, a complex set of rules and interpretations is issued by the intermediary. As the largest intermediary, Blue Cross has issued more letters and instructions than other intermediaries, such as Aetna or Mutual of Omaha. Therefore, there has been more opportunity for individual interpretation with those other intermediaries. They have not faced as many situations as Blue Cross has and have been able to interpret regulations more often in favor of the hospital.

Until the 1980s, this advantage was very significant. Blue Cross was clearly the least desirable choice as an intermediary. Now, however, the regulations from HCFA are so rigid and so comprehensive that they overshadow interpretations promulgated by the intermediary. There is very little room for interpretation left to the intermediary today. Thus, the desirability of other intermediaries over Blue Cross is no longer as significant.

A small percentage of hospitals have chosen to deal directly with HHS and have elected not to have an intermediary. Without an intermediary, the Social Security Administration is responsible for the audit of the cost report. However, the Social Security Administration reportedly either does no audit or subcontracts the audit to small accounting firms with no Medicare knowledge. The advantage, therefore, of not having an intermediary is in the absence of an annual audit. Any hospital that is considering this option should be aware that the advantage involved could rapidly disappear. At this writing, however, those few hospitals who have elected to deal directly with the Social Security Administration usually have the advantage of no annual audit or a very weak audit.

Viewpoint of the Intermediary

It is important to note that the intermediaries have a viewpoint that is different from that of the providers. This is due to the fact that they are paid to reduce reimbursement to providers, and also to the fact that they are taught to respect the health insurance manuals, intermediary letters, rulings, and other similar data. Providers attempt to increase reimbursement and are not bound by any rules or regulations beyond those promulgated by the HHS. Therefore, disputes, controversies, and appeals should be expected.

Figure 3–2 illustrates the phenomenon of different viewpoints. It is a picture of a woman. Before looking at it, be prepared to answer these two questions:

1. Is the woman over 50 years old?
2. Would I trust her?

Half of the persons looking at this picture will see a young woman, and half will see an old woman. Similarly, half of the persons looking at this picture will want to trust the woman, and half will not trust her. In a large group, there would be an argument over which was the correct choice.

In fact, there is both an old woman and a young woman in Figure 3–2. All of a person's mental tapes contribute to determining which woman he or she sees. A person's childhood experiences, schools, occupations, friends, and acquaintances all contribute to what that person sees when looking at the picture. There is no right or wrong answer; there are just different or opposing answers.

In the same way, Medicare auditors have views that are different from those of hospital financial personnel. The different views are neither right nor wrong, correct nor incorrect; they are merely different because of different backgrounds. Still, it would be totally inappropriate for hospital personnel to rely upon Blue Cross or other intermediaries for Medicare expertise. This applies as well to Medicaid, Blue Cross, and other cost reports. Many hospitals recognize the good faith effort of intermediaries

Figure 3–2 Picture of a Woman

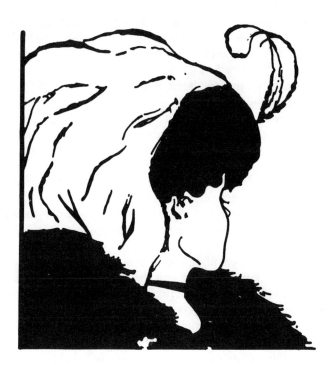

to obtain additional reimbursement or to interpret regulations on behalf of the hospitals, and they believe they are thereby maximizing reimbursement. But those hospitals that rely solely on their intermediaries may be losing thousands of dollars in allowable reimbursement. The intermediary auditors normally do everything they can see to assist hospitals; however, their vision is clouded by rules that the hospitals can ignore.

THE APPEAL PROCESS

The Intermediary Appeal Process

All intermediaries are required to grant hearings on disputes that involve between $1,000 and $10,000 in reimbursement. Disputes involving $10,000 or more are heard exclusively by the PRRB. If it is difficult to determine whether there is $1,000 or more reimbursement in dispute, the intermediary must resolve the dispute in favor of the provider.

After the audit has been completed, the intermediary must send the provider an official document called the notice of program reimbursement. In this notice, the intermediary:

- explains the amount due the hospital or due the program
- shows how this amount differs from the filed cost report
- explains the differences, giving references
- informs the hospital of its right to appeal if the appeal is made within 180 days from the date of the notice of program reimbursement.

Often, the intermediary will cite rulings, manual sections, bureau policy, intermediary letters, or other references for proposed audit adjustments. Since the hospital is not bound by these, it should insist that the intermediary cite the applicable section of the law or the regulation of the secretary of HHS.

The notice of program reimbursement is a very important document because it is the foundation upon which the appeal must be based. Very few notices adequately cite the proper reference. Often audit adjustments cite a reference in HIM–15 or make a general statement to support the adjustments. The hospital should insist on a properly documented reference for all such audit adjustments. If the intermediary does not comply and a sufficient amount of money is in dispute, the hospital should consider taking the matter to the courts. The hospital has a right to know which regulation is being used to support the proposed adjustment; it is not bound by anything beyond the regulations.

After receiving the notice of program reimbursement, the hospital has 180 days in which to request a hearing. The request, which must be in writing, should state which proposed audit adjustments are being disputed, should explain why the hospital objects to the adjustments, and should include documentation to support the dispute. Requests for a hearing can be made after the 180-day deadline, but the intermediary is not required to comply with such requests. Depending upon the circumstances, the complexity of the case, or other factors, the intermediary may deny a request for a hearing that is made after the 180 days. The intermediary is not allowed to reopen a cost report if more than three years have transpired since the notice of program reimbursement.

The provider can file a request for a hearing any time after receiving the notice of program reimbursement. However, if there is a chance that the dispute can be settled with the auditors, the request for a hearing should be delayed as long as possible. Once a request has been filed, the matter can no longer be resolved by the auditors. The only person who can resolve a dispute once the hearing has been requested is the hearing officer. Most of the time, if the auditors and the provider reach an agreement before the hearing, the matter will be dropped by the hearing officer, but the latter is not compelled to do this.

Often, Blue Cross will attempt to schedule the intermediary appeal hearing in Chicago. The provider has a right to ask that the hearing be held at a more convenient place. If requested, the hearing can be at the office of the provider's local intermediary or at some other convenient place.

In preparation for the hearing, the provider should request a "prehearing discovery." This is a meeting with the local intermediary in which the hospital or other provider reviews audit workpapers, correspondence, and other data that the auditors have gathered. Often the intermediary will not share all of the data in its files. This is especially true of surveys. However, it should be noted that, in a field audit, the intermediary has access to most of the hospital's records. If the intermediary withholds some data and the hospital believes that the data are important, the provider can seek court action.

Just before the hearing, it is recommended that the provider have a conference with the intermediary. At this meeting, the points in dispute as well as the points agreed upon can be finalized. Also, any last-minute preparations can be made. This is the last chance to reach agreement before the hearing.

The hearing is held either by a panel of three hearing officers or by a single hearing officer. Most of the time, the hearing is held by a single hearing officer. The hearing is between the hearing officer and the provider; the local Blue Cross plan or other local intermediary is not included. Of course, the hearing officer has information supplied by the intermediary, including questions to ask the provider.

There are both advantages and disadvantages to not having the intermediary present as part of the hearing. However, the disadvantages outweigh the advantages. The main disadvantage is that the provider cannot cross-examine, dispute, or ask questions concerning material provided by the intermediary because the intermediary is not present.

Often, as we have noted, the Blue Cross intermediary hearing is scheduled at the Blue Cross offices in Chicago. The provider is informed of its right to waive a personal appearance at the hearing. Without a personal appearance, the hearing is decided solely on the basis of the written material that is presented. Because of the expense involved in traveling to Chicago, many providers waive their right to a personal appearance. In fact, it may be better to insist on a hearing in a city more convenient to the provider than to waive the right to a personal appearance at the hearing. Blue Cross may resist this request because of the time and expense involved in sending a hearing officer to the provider's site. However, a hospital administrator's time is just as valuable as that of a Blue Cross hearing officer. Thus, the hospital should insist on a convenient site if its presence at the hearing will make a significant difference.

At the hearing, the provider presents its evidence and is questioned by the hearing officer. Then the intermediary's position is presented, and the provider is allowed to ask questions. After the hearing, the panel or hearing officer renders a decision. That decision is subject to review by the Bureau of Health Insurance (BHI). In this context, it is important to note that the hearing officer is bound by all relevant health insurance manuals, intermediary letters, bulletins, program policies, and general instructions. But, as noted earlier, the hospital or other provider is not bound by these. Predictably, therefore, most cases that are heard in the intermediary appeal process are decided in favor of the intermediary and against the provider.

The decision of the hearing officer is final. There are no provisions in the Medicare program for appealing the decision. Since the intermediary appeal process is used only for disputes involving less than $10,000 of reimbursement, it would not normally be cost effective for the provider to attempt additional actions.

Thus, the intermediary appeal process is heavily weighted in favor of the intermediary. For this reason, it is often advantageous for a hospital to contact several other hospitals or other providers and to plan a group appeal through the PRRB. To be considered by the PRRB, the group appeal must involve at least $50,000 in additional reimbursement. If the PRRB renders an adverse opinion, the matter can be taken to a U.S. district court. An appeal through these channels is expensive, but the chances of eventually winning are incalculably better than through the provider appeal process. Also, it should be noted that in a group appeal the expenses are shared by several providers, making the process more affordable.

The Provider Reimbursement Review Board

The PRRB, as we have noted, has jurisdiction over disputes in which the amount of additional reimbursement involved is $10,000 or more. On group appeals, the amount in controversy must be $50,000 or more, and the question of law or fact must be identical for all of the providers in the group appeal.

The PRRB was created in legislation passed in 1972, but it was not established until 1974. The board consists of five members who are appointed to three-year terms by the secretary of HHS. At least one member of the board must be a certified public accountant. It takes a quorum of at least three members, one of whom must be a certified public accountant, to hear a case. The chairman is the only member of the board who is a full-time government employee. The board meets in Baltimore, Maryland.

Hearings before the PRRB are adversarial in nature. Both the intermediary and the provider present evidence, cross-examine, and introduce witnesses. The hearings are very similar to court proceedings. The board can even issue subpoenas. Because of the nature of a PRRB hearing, it is important that the hospital or other provider retain in advance legal counsel as well as a certified public accountant who is an expert in Medicare reimbursement.

The legal and professional fees for a PRRB hearing at this writing average approximately $20,000 to $30,000. In addition, there are travel and other expenses involved. If the case is then appealed to a district court, the provider will spend an additional $10,000 to $15,000. Because of this high cost, as we have noted, it is often advantageous to file a group appeal with other hospitals that have the same issue in dispute. In a group appeal, the costs are shared by all parties. The costs can also be reduced by using a hospital's local attorney and local certified public accounting firm, but normally the chances of winning are thereby significantly reduced.

Preparation for a PRRB hearing is similar to that for an intermediary hearing. The provider files a request for an appeal, which contains the following items:

- the cost report year that is being contested
- the date of the notice of program reimbursement
- the adjustment or adjustments that are being contested
- a one- or two-paragraph summary of the provider's position
- the reason why the provider believes the adjustment is inaccurate

Once the request for a hearing has been made and the PRRB has accepted jurisdiction over the matter, the provider must act quickly. A request should be sent to the BHI under the Freedom of Information Act, requesting any information that bureau has on the issue. Letters of bureau policy, memoranda, workpapers, and other relevant data should be requested. The intermediary should be asked to provide its specific reason for the disallowance. Meetings should be scheduled with the intermediary to obtain agreement on some issues, thereby reducing the points in dispute.

The provider should have several issues in the appeal. Because the costs of the appeal are approximately the same with several points in dispute as with only one point in dispute, the additional issues are free. Having several issues in the appeal allows the PRRB to rule at least partially in favor of both parties.

As prehearing discovery meetings are held with the intermediary, the BHI should be gathering documents underlying its policy in response to the request via the Freedom of Information Act. The bureau maintains a file on every manual of instruction, so this should not take too long. Often the information received will contain documents to support the provider's position. For this reason, it may be beneficial to request information on a particular policy relating to adjustments that the provider will not appeal to the PRRB, as well as information on those that will be appealed.

If the hearing is scheduled before the provider's case is complete, the provider should request an extension. Extensions are often granted to provide time to make the presentation clearer. Often, the provider and the intermediary are able to resolve the issue before the PRRB hearing. In this case, the board can be requested to dismiss the issue.

At a PRRB hearing, the intermediary often presents new arguments or new evidence. Since the provider has asked for all the evidence in the prehearing discovery, the attorney or certified public accountant should make it clear at the hearing that the presented evidence is new.

PRRB Decisions

It is clear from its charter that the PRRB is not bound by BHI policy, health insurance manuals (HIM–10 or HIM–15), intermediary letters, general instructions, or other pronouncements. It is instructed to give great weight to all of this material, yet it rules in favor of the intermediary more often than it rules in favor of the provider. This is predictable, especially when one considers that the research staff that supports the board is comprised of full-time government employees and that the five members of the board are appointed by the secretary of HHS.

The secretary of HHS has the authority to modify or reverse the decisions of the PRRB. In normal practice, only decisions favorable to the provider are modified or reversed. The secretary's authority must be exercised within 60 days of the date of the decision. After 60 days, the decision of the board can be changed only by the courts.

When an adverse decision is received, the hospital should immediately summarize the "suggested findings" in a letter to the PRRB. The summary should contain references, interpretations, and other relevant data. The purpose of the summary is to help uphold the hospital's position in the event the dispute is appealed in federal court. Therefore, it should be designed to support the hospital's case. This summary is included in the legal brief that is filed with the appeal.

Court Appeals

If the provider is not satisfied with the ruling of the PRRB as amended by the secretary, it can file a complaint in a federal district court. The hospital has a choice of filing in the district court where it is located or in the District of Columbia. Normally it is better to file in the hospital's home district. Historically, the home district courts have been more favorable to the providers than the District of Columbia court. The complaint must be filed within 60 days of the decision by the PRRB or the secretary of HHS.

The district court trial does not involve witnesses, cross-examinations, and attorneys. A set of briefs is prepared to summarize the positions. No new evidence is introduced beyond that introduced at the PRRB hearing. For this reason, the evidence presented at the PRRB hearing should be as complete as possible.

The district court usually denies oral arguments. The decision arrives by mail after the judge has completed deliberations. Hospitals and other providers normally do very well in the district courts. Unlike the intermediary appeal process and the PRRB, the district courts normally give providers their proportionate share of favorable judgments. On nearly all district court cases where it loses, the government appeals to a higher court. The higher court is bound only by the regulations promulgated by the secretary; it does not consider bureau policy, intermediary letters, health insurance manuals, or other similar documentation.

AVOIDING APPEALS

Advance Rulings

The provider can request an advance ruling from either the intermediary or the district office of the HCFA. There is no formal process for either of these requests. Normally, a well-organized letter with attachments to clarify the issues is sent and an opinion is requested. Advance rulings are relatively easy to obtain. If the ruling is favorable to the provider, it can be used to support the handling of that particular issue on the cost report. If the ruling is not favorable to the provider, there is no requirement to follow it. However, if the provider does not follow the ruling, it must be prepared to appeal the issue.

The Field Audit

If the provider makes proper preparation for the field audit and manages it as much as possible, controversies can be reduced. Before the field audit takes place, the provider should ask the intermediary's director of auditing how much time has been budgeted for it. Then the provider should identify all the gray issues in the cost report, noting those that could result in significant audit adjustments and those that would not. It is to the provider's advantage to have the auditors look at those areas where adjustments, if any, would be minimal. Conversely, the provider should be aware of those areas in which significant adverse adjustments might be made by the audit. The provider's objective is, of course, to avoid significant adjustments.

Medicare auditors and other cost report auditors should not be allowed to talk with department directors or administrative staff members without a member of the controller's staff present. This is true for follow-up phone calls as well as for meetings during the field audit. A Medicare auditor may ask a department director how much effort a particular task requires; and the director, perhaps a bit tired and frustrated, might reply, "That takes half of my time." The statement may not be accurate, but it could still be used to support an adverse cost calculation. This is only one example of the type of adverse effect that may result when auditors talk with department directors. For such reasons, department directors should be instructed to ask the auditors to direct all questions to a member of the controller's staff.

Similarly, during the field audit, the auditors should not be allowed to use the provider's photocopy equipment. Instead, a person in the business office should be assigned to make all required photocopies for the auditors. A log should be maintained of all material photocopied at the request of Medicare auditors. In this way, the controller knows exactly what information has been given to the auditors.

It is important to remember that, during the audit process, providers are not required to release to the auditors all the information they request. Only that information that is needed to make a fair determination of potential liability must be shared with the auditors. This does not necessarily include everything they ask for. To clarify this point, let us look at a couple of examples.

Often the Medicare auditors will ask to review the minutes of the provider's board of directors. However, such board minutes should not be shared with Medicare auditors, even if there is nothing in them that could someday be used as a basis for an adverse audit adjustment. At some future time, those minutes could contain more sensitive material, and a precedent of sharing would have been established.

At times, the auditors may learn of a special study or analysis that the hospital has completed and ask to see a copy. The hospital should use extreme care in such a situation. Normally, special analyses, consultants' reports, long-range plans, comparative data, and other such information of a nonroutine nature should not be shared with Medicare and Medicaid auditors. In short, when the auditors ask for a piece of information, the provider should consider whether it is relevant and whether it could result in an adverse audit adjustment before providing it.

Throughout the field audit, the controller or reimbursement expert should attempt to stay informed. Regular meetings should be held with the auditors to determine how the audit is going and to inquire about proposed audit adjustments. Although adverse audit adjustments should be strongly resisted, the controller should remain cordial toward the auditors, should take them to lunch, be friendly, and appear helpful. Many proposed audit adjustments are made at the discretion of the field auditors. If the provider firmly resists adverse adjustments yet has been cooperative, the adjustments are likely to be fewer in number.

Small adjustments are to be expected; the provider should not quarrel over insignificant issues. If the intermediary becomes upset, the audit may well become more detailed and the posture of the auditor more demanding. It is important to maintain good relations with the auditors.

The Exit Conference

After the field audit, the intermediary will determine the proposed audit adjustments and ask for an exit conference to discuss them. The provider should insist upon enough time to study the proposed adjustments prior to the exit conference. Two to three weeks is a reasonable period. In any case, the provider should not agree to an exit conference without adequate time to study the proposed adjustments. Sometimes, the intermediary will want to present the adjustments for the first time at the exit conference. In such cases, it should be noted that the intermediary has had several months to research the proposed adjustments and that the provider has every right to review them in advance of the exit conference.

Blue Cross, the regional office of HCFA, and other entities can direct the local intermediary to make certain adjustments. In addition, the intermediary is bound by a set of rules that the provider is not bound by. This is important to remember when reviewing proposed adjustments.

In preparation for the exit conference, the provider should review the photocopy log showing the material the auditors used during the field audit and also the progress notes made during the audit. This will help the hospital understand the basis for the proposed adjustments. In addition, the provider should read the cited regulations for all significant adjustments. Through such careful preparation, many disputes can be eliminated during the exit conference.

At the conference, each proposed adverse adjustment should be discussed. Although this is not the final opportunity to dispute the intermediary's findings, beyond the exit conference the context becomes more formal and the process is more closely defined. Therefore, it is to the hospital's advantage to settle disputes in the exit conference or at least prepare the groundwork at this meeting for future appeals.

Setting a Posture

One of the most important things a hospital or other provider can do to minimize appeals is to establish the proper posture. Many proposed audit adjustments involve gray areas, for the intermediary as well as for the provider. If the auditor and the provider have established a cordial, yet business-like, relationship, there will be fewer adjustments.

If the hospital is too aggressive on insignificant matters, the auditor may make excessive adjustments. If the hospital is abrasive in its opposition to proposed adjustments, the auditor may be less willing to compromise. In short, the provider should be aggressive, yet willing to compromise. The negotiations should be firm, yet not abrasive.

Chapter 4

Accounting Techniques

There are certain accounting techniques that have proven successful in maximizing Medicare reimbursement. These techniques are not applicable to all institutions, and they are not all-inclusive; but, as shown in this and subsequent chapters, they illustrate a way of thinking that can maximize reimbursement. (Current Medicare forms and instructions pertaining to accounting techniques are contained in Appendix B. These should be reviewed in conjunction with this chapter to gain a better understanding of the relevant techniques.)

GENERAL LEDGER EXPENSES

Since general ledger expenses are the starting point for Medicare, they represent a solid base upon which the hospital can maximize Medicare reimbursement.

Timing of Maximization Techniques

It is important to apply Medicare maximization techniques as early in the accounting process as possible. It is best if a technique can be applied monthly as part of the normal general ledger process. This is not always possible, however, because it may confuse department directors and render monthly variance reporting meaningless. The second best time to apply such techniques—to make allocations, reclassifications, and other general ledger adjustments—is at year end, between the preliminary trial balance and the final trial balance, when the hospital makes most of its year-end closing entries and financial statements, including the final department budget reports, are prepared and distributed. These statements are used to judge performance. The journal entries at this point can reclassify expenses from one department to another, apportion expenses, and affect other Medicare maximization techniques. After these final closing entries are made, a final trial balance of expenses is prepared. This is the trial balance that is given to the Medicare auditors and the hospital's independent outside auditors.

Often a hospital makes reclassifications and apportionments that it does not want included as part of its audited financial statements. These techniques are applied solely to maximize reimbursement. Perhaps the technique is not based on GAAP, or it is not consistent with past financial reporting. As stated earlier, Medicare cost reports do not always follow GAAP. In these cases, most of the reclassifications, apportionments, and other such accounting techniques should be made on an accounting workpaper rather than on the Medicare cost report. This is true even if there is a place on the cost report schedules to accommodate the application of the technique.

Adjustments that are made on the cost report forms are part of the cost report process. These are relatively easy for Medicare auditors to disallow because it is only necessary to show that they are not allowed by Medicare principles. Adjustments that are made prior to completing the cost report forms are part of the hospital's accounting process, which is governed by GAAP.

GAAP are promulgated by the American Institute of Certified Public Accountants, the Financial Accounting Standards Board, the American Accounting Association, and other such groups. Although the Medicare program is not governed by GAAP, their auditors must cite a specific regulation to reverse something that is incorporated as part of the hospital's accounting process. The hospital has a stronger position in potential appeal processes if something is recorded as part of its accounting process rather than as part of its Medicare process.

As noted in Chapter 3, disputes with Medicare auditors are likely to occur because the latter are bound by rules that are different from those that govern hospitals. Thus, it is important to build a strong base from which to defend the hospital's position in such disputes. By positioning maximization techniques early in the accounting process, the hospital's position is strengthened.

Additions to Costs

As we have seen, the Medicare and Medicaid programs are not administered according to GAAP. Most of the deviations from those principles reduce reimbursement. The techniques discussed in this section represent additions to costs as determined by Medicare principles. Not all of these techniques represent GAAP.

Hospitals and other providers have some costs that can be added to general ledger costs for Medicare. The first such costs to determine are those that represent services of a related organization. If the provider is a county hospital and the county removes snow from the driveways, dumps stone or sand, provides administrative support, or provides any other service, the hospital should impute a cost for the service and add it to the cost report. It is not significant that the hospital is not charged for the service. Costs associated with approving the annual budget, setting policies, or obtaining financing can also be considered for inclusion in the cost report.

If the hospital is part of a religious order or other chain, any service provided by the mother house or home office should be added for cost report purposes. State hospitals often have certain purchases made for them at the state capitol; these costs should be added. The hospital's position is also strengthened if it writes checks to pay for such services, but this is not essential.

Another cost that can be added, but is often overlooked, is volunteer help. If a hospital volunteer works at least 20 hours per week in a position that would require a paid employee, the hospital can impute a reasonable salary plus a fringe benefit amount that can be added to cost. In order to claim volunteer services, there must be an obligation on the part of the volunteer to continue performing the service. In cases where the hospital can project future reimbursement for applicable volunteers, the volunteers' obligation to continue performing the service may be procured. When the volunteers wish to discontinue the work, the hospital can relieve them of the obligation. Agreements of this kind are not normally enforceable, but they still can be used to increase reimbursement.

Depreciation is allowed on donated assets. This includes assets purchased by the state, county, and other related organizations. It also includes assets donated by organizations, vendors, physicians, and others. It is often difficult to capitalize donated assets because the fixed asset ledger is updated from the hospital's accounts payable system. It is important, however, to create an awareness throughout the hospital that donated assets represent an opportunity for additional cost reimbursement. All donations should be reported to the accounting department. These assets can then be depreciated.

Fund Accounting

Under certain circumstances, expenditures made from funds other than the general fund can be included on the cost report. These include certain expenditures from grant funds or donated funds. Normally, however, grant fund and donated fund expenditures are not included. If the hospital does not have separate funds, then expenditures made out of the general fund that would appropriately be included in other funds are excluded from the cost report.

Expenses from restricted grants are not allowed for Medicare unless the grant is specifically classified as a seed money grant. Organizations and agencies that provide grants are often not aware of these Medicare implications. The hospital should resist the application of restrictions on grant funds. Unrestricted grant funds can be used to pay expenses for a project that are allowable on the cost report. The hospital, in effect, receives payment twice: once from the grant source, and again from Medicare and Medicaid. If an organization will not agree to an unrestricted grant, the hospital should request that the grant document specifically identify the funds as a seed money grant.

Donated funds are treated the same as grant funds for purposes of Medicare and Medicaid. The hospital should, therefore, attempt to have all donations given to the institution without restrictions. Restricted donations are offset against expenses for cost report purposes; unrestricted donations are used to pay expenses, which are allowable costs. As with unrestricted grants, the hospital is paid twice. If the hospital cannot obtain an unrestricted donation and part of the donated funds will be used to purchase fixed assets, the donor should be asked to purchase the assets rather than donate the money. As previously noted, depreciation can be taken on the cost reports for donated assets. Having the donor purchase the fixed assets is the only way to receive reimbursement for restricted gifts.

ADJUSTMENTS TO EXPENSES

It is important to remember that most of the adjustments to expenses required for Medicare and Medicaid are not based on GAAP. Such adjustments should not, therefore, be made on Blue Cross cost reports, on cost reports with other payers, on submissions to rate-setting agencies, or on schedules used to support rate increases, unless specifically required by contract or regulation with the relevant organization.

Depreciation

Many of the assets used by the hospital may be fully depreciated. This is common in all industries. If the hospital can identify fully depreciated assets that were purchased prior to the Medicare program (1967), the lives of these assets can be extended to recoup additional reimbursement. This shifts excess depreciation taken in pre-Medicare years into the Medicare years. This technique is normally applied on a workpaper rather than on the actual fixed asset ledger. In this way, the published accounting records do not need to be restated, and the computerized fixed asset records do not have to be adjusted.

The various components of a building should be depreciated separately in order to maximize reimbursement. This allows the hospital to recover its capital costs more rapidly. If the elevators need to be replaced before the building is torn down, the costs associated with the elevators should be broken out and depreciated separately. Since roofs seldom last more than 20 years, they can be depreciated separately. Other components of a building that can be depreciated separately include the plumbing, heating and air conditioning, electrical components, and fixtures.

When planning the construction of a new building or wing, it is desirable to request the contractor to determine construction costs per square feet by department. In square feet, radiology and surgery are much more expensive to construct than routine care. In turn, routine care construction is more expensive than pathology construction. If the hospital has determined construction costs per square feet by department and the departments with high construction costs are also relatively highly cost reimbursed, the hospital can use this information to maximize reimbursement. If this information does not benefit the hospital, it need not be used.

When a provider leaves the Medicare or Medicaid program, the intermediary is required to recoup any amount that represents the difference between straight-line depreciation and accelerated depreciation methods. Accelerated depreciation was allowed until August 1970. Although recouping of this depreciation is required in the Medicare regulations, it has been held to be unconstitutional by the courts under the Fifth Amendment. The courts found that the original regulations contained neither qualifications for using accelerated depreciation nor provisions for recapturing the costs. The use of retroactive regulations was determined to be a violation of the hospital's right to due process.

Reclassifications

There are two types of reclassifications—those required by the Medicare program, and those elected by the hospital to maximize reimbursement. In this section we discuss only those reclassifications elected by the hospital to maximize reimbursement. (Instructions pertaining to those required by Medicare are included in Appendix B.) Reclassifications to increase reimbursement should always be made as part of the hospital's accounting process. These should not be made on the cost report schedules.

Before reclassifications can be determined, a ranking schedule must be studied. A typical ranking schedule is illustrated in Table 4–1. In this example, for every $1.00 of cost in coronary care, Community Hospital receives $.85; and for every $1.00 of cost in a private room, the hospital receives $.32. If the hospital can reallocate $100 from the private room cost center to coronary care, it will receive an additional $53 in reimbursement. If the hospital can reallocate $100 from physical therapy to respiratory therapy, it will receive an additional $30 in reimbursement.

The objective of cost reclassification is to reclassify costs into a higher cost reimbursed department unless the reimbursement in the higher ranked department is limited by a ceiling or limit. For example, if routine care is higher cost reimbursed than the ancillaries, costs should be shifted into routine care.

It should be noted that reclassifications may be challenged vigorously by the Medicare intermediary. Therefore, these adjustments should be supported by documentation, cost studies, and schedules. In addition, it should be expected that the hospital may not have all of the reclassifications allowed, and the appeal process may at times cost more than the benefit derived.

The following represent opportunities for possible reclassifications:

- In some hospitals the nurses do the IV admixtures. This is a pharmacy function. Therefore, part of nursing costs can be given to pharmacy.

Table 4–1 Community Hospital Ranking Schedule

		Percentage of Revenue That Is:	
Revenue Center	Rank	Charge Reimbursed	Cost Reimbursed
Private room	30	68%	32%
↓	↓	↓	↓
Nuclear medicine	6	61	39
Physical therapy	5	50	50
Laboratory	4	45	55
Intensive care	3	30	70
Respiratory care	2	20	80
Coronary care	1	15	85

- Nursing personnel normally ask for urine samples and sometimes draw blood samples. These are pathology functions. Therefore, part of these nursing costs can be given to the laboratory.
- Dietary nourishments can be part of routine or remain part of dietary; if they remain in dietary, a part of this cost will be reallocated to cafeteria.
- Emergency room personnel often perform admitting functions. Therefore, part of the emergency room cost can be given to the business office.
- There may be cashiers in the cafeteria, clinics, emergency room, and other departments. Therefore, part of these department costs can be given to the business office.
- Costs associated with transporting inpatients to the ancillary departments for treatment can be reclassified to the ancillaries if the service is performed by nursing service personnel, or they can be reclassified to routine service if the service is performed by ancillary department personnel.

The potential for reclassification is almost unlimited. To take advantage of this technique, it is recommended that the controller review the entire general ledger at least once a year with a ranking schedule. This should be done in a quiet place away from the office, and at least two days should be allotted to the task. Account by account, the controller should ask if there is another department to which the expenses can be reclassified to receive additional reimbursement. Each time this exercise is performed, new potentials for additional reimbursement will be identified.

Offsets and Adjustments

Medicare regulations require that all "other operating and nonoperating" sources of income be offset against expenses for Medicare. This reduces allowable costs and, therefore, reduces cost reimbursement. To illustrate this principle, assume that the housekeeping department incurs $100,000 of expenses for the year. Assume further that revenue from cot rental is $5,000 for the year. Medicare regulations require that the cot rental income be offset against the cost of the housekeeping department. Thus:

Cost of housekeeping department	$100,000
Less income from cot rental	5,000
Housekeeping costs for Medicare	$ 95,000

For the Medicare cost report, the hospital would record the housekeeping department expenses as $95,000, notwithstanding the fact that the real cost was $100,000. This offset reduces the Medicare allowable expenses and ultimately Medicare reimbursement.

In each applicable instance, the regulations require the hospital to offset either cash received or cost, if cost can be determined. The regulations allow the hospital to make a profit without compromise if the profit can be determined. Costs are normally significantly less than cash received. These adjustments are made on Schedule A–8. The hospital should perform a cost analysis on every A–8 offset. If costs are less than cash received, this should be used for the required adjustment against expenses. If costs are greater than cash received, cash should be used for the required adjustment against expenses.

Following are several costing techniques that can be used to minimize these offsets and adjustments:

- As we have noted, cot rental must be offset against housekeeping. To determine the cost of cot rental service, a cost study is performed. The greatest portion of these costs is personnel time. The cost accountant performs a time study on personnel when the cots are taken to the patient room and set up. The accountant should watch the time carefully when doing the study, thereby making the housekeeping personnel aware of the time involved in a nonthreatening way. As a result, the cot is placed in the room relatively quickly, yet there is still a valid cost study. When it is time to take the cot down and prepare it for the next person, the accountant again carefully records the time. The cot is returned to storage and stored quickly, because the housekeeping personnel are aware of the fact they are being timed. In order to further reduce the time involved, this cost study should be scheduled for a time when the elevators are not likely to be in use by others. In this way, the time spent waiting for elevators is kept to a minimum.
- Hospitals normally grant one photographer the exclusive right to take pictures of babies in the nursery. For this, the hospital may receive several thousand dollars in royalties from the photographer. The hospital can determine that these royalties represent unrestricted donations and not offset this income on the cost reports. Another strategy is to offset a cost of $12 on the cost report. This assumes that it costs $1.00 per month to accept and deposit the check from the photographer.
- Medical records abstracts are customarily sold for $10 to $20 apiece. When costed out properly, the cost is about $2.00 in most hospitals. The cost accountant asks medical records personnel to gather several abstracts for a cost study. Doing several at one time is more efficient

than doing them one at a time, so the cost will be lower. The cost accountant watches the time as the abstracts are prepared. When employees are being timed, they work relatively faster. Yet, with several observations, this is still a valid cost study. An amount is added for postage, supplies, and copy expense to complete the study.

- Hospitals normally receive rebates from the telephone company because of pay telephones on the premises. As with other income, either the cash received or the cost must be offset against expenses on the cost report. The only expense associated with pay telephones is the time spent by housekeeping personnel to wipe them off occasionally. This expense is minimal and normally significantly less than cash received.

- Vending machines are normally very profitable. The main costs associated with vending machines are electricity and the cost of keeping them clean. The amount of electricity can be determined with a meter. Many vending machines use no electricity at all. The cost of keeping vending machines clean must be determined by a cost study.

- Most hospitals rent television sets to patients by the day. Depreciation and maintenance of these sets are relatively easy to estimate with a simple cost study. If the hospital places a meter on one of the sets, the amount of kilowatts used per hour can be determined. The hospital purchases electricity at a low rate per kilowatt hour because it is a large user. Most hospitals pay ten cents or less for the electricity to run a television set for eight hours. Eight hours is a reasonable estimate of the amount of time a patient watches television in an average day. If the television service is provided by an independent agency with the hospital receiving royalties, the only cost incurred by the hospital is the ten cents per day or less for electricity.

- Many utility companies have a graduated rate for kilowatts used. As more electricity is consumed, the rate charged per kilowatt hour decreases. Hospitals with a graduated rate should use the lowest rate to calculate the cost of electricity used for vending machines and patient television service. This assumes that these are not essential services and, therefore, should be charged at the rate for the lowest amount of kilowatts used. Some intermediaries will not agree with this viewpoint. In such cases, since it does not in any case represent a significant amount of money, the hospital can concede and use the average rate charged, but only if the intermediary concedes a different point that results in as much or more reimbursement.

- If the hospital recovers silver from old radiology films, the cost of the silver should be determined. Silver prices have increased dramatically in recent years. Therefore, cash received is normally significantly more than cost for silver.

It is not possible to cite all of the possible Schedule A–8 adjustments for all hospitals. However, the above examples illustrate the principle that in these adjustments, almost without exception, the cost is less than cash received. Thus the hospital should carefully study every Schedule A–8 adjustment. With careful planning, a cost study can be performed to determine cost. These studies should be planned to minimize the amount of cost that must be offset.

The intermediary auditor may challenge some of these cost studies or disallow the adjustment on cost rather than on cash received. Their challenges may be in response to an intermediary letter, a specific policy instruction from the regional office of the HCFA, a section of the health insurance manuals, a provider letter, or some other document. The hospital, however, is not bound by any of these. The hospital should always insist that the intermediary cite the applicable regulation. A firm stand should be taken with the intermediary if the regulation can be interpreted to the hospital's advantage. If the regulation does not specifically exclude an accounting technique, the hospital can assume a right to use it.

COST ACCOUNTING

Accounting is an art rather than a science. For every required accounting action, the accountant can choose any one of several GAAP. This section presents several cost accounting techniques that have been used to maximize reimbursement.

Patient Telephone Cost

The Medicare Bureau has ruled that patient telephone costs are not patient care related. The intermediaries have been instructed to disallow these costs. The reasons cited are being challenged by the hospital industry. Individual hospitals should not offset patient telephone cost even though the intermediary is required to make an adjustment for this. However, the hospital should calculate the cost of patient telephones and give the results to the intermediary. In this manner, the hospital protects its position and at the same time provides documentation to reduce the amount of disallowed cost.

The determination of the amount of cost associated with patient telephones begins with an operator peg count. For a defined period of time, the hospital switchboard operators count the number of patient-related calls and the number of nonpatient-related calls handled. The amount of time spent on patient-related calls will be disallowed. The hospital should carefully plan the time of the peg count. The count should always be performed during a period of low census so that the number of patient calls will be minimal. To accomplish this, the hospital first identifies a low census month. Then a time within that month is chosen. If the intermediary allows a three- or four-day peg count study, the days chosen should be near the end of the week. Normally, the patient census is lower near the end of the week than at the beginning of the week. Use of the latter part of a week still results in a valid cost study, but it skews the results in favor of the hospital.

Hospital telephone calls normally take significantly more operator time than do patient telephone calls. The reasons for this include the placing of long-distance calls for departments, paging of personnel, responding to emergencies, and waiting for answers when departments are away from the telephone. A time study will determine how much more operator time is spent on hospital-related calls. This time study should be conducted during that part of the week or day when the number of paging and long distance calls is highest. The results of the peg count are thus weighted to reduce the percentage of time spent on patient-related calls.

Only the salary of switchboard operators during the time patients can receive calls should be included. Patients normally cannot receive calls during the night. However, if the hospital has direct-dial patient phone service, no part of the switchboard operator's time should be allocated to patient calls.

A third technique used to reduce the offset for patient telephones is to study the number of calls made by physicians, nursing personnel, and other hospital personnel from patient telephones. The study can also determine how many times the patient used the telephone to call hospital departments, make physician appointments, inquire about insurance coverage, and make other patient care related calls. It is not uncommon to find that 20 to 25 percent of the calls made from patient telephones are patient care related. That portion of the patient telephone cost should not be included in the amount disallowed.

With careful planning, the amount of costs ultimately offset as nonpatient care related will be an insignificant portion of the base telephone equipment cost, plus operator time. Long-distance expense is not included in this allocation because it is 100-percent patient care related and therefore allowed.

Capital Costs

There is an opportunity for additional reimbursement on capital purchases in which the vendor offers a warranty or training. The hospital should request that the cost of the warranty, as well as the cost of all vendor training of hospital personnel in the use of the new equipment, be itemized separately on the invoice for new equipment. These amounts can then be expensed immediately rather than capitalized and depreciated over the useful life of the equipment. This allows the hospital to recover its cost more rapidly. On purchases of complex equipment that requires several days of offsite training, this can be a significant amount. Vendors that are not accustomed to breaking out the cost of training and warranty on capital invoices should make an estimate. If the purpose of requiring the estimate is explained, vendors often list a relatively large proportion of the total purchase price to training and warranty in order to benefit the hospital.

The hospital should review its capitalization policy on a regular basis. In a tax-exempt hospital, it is to the hospital's advantage to expense as many purchases as possible, consistent with GAAP. Adding machines, calculators, small equipment items, file cabinets, dietary utensils, and other like items should be expensed in the year of purchase. In a for-profit hospital, the controller must calculate the benefits of federal investment tax credits, rapid write-off of equipment under President Reagan's tax reform measures, and return on equity. For-profit hospitals will often capitalize small equipment items.

Remodeling and renovations can often be either expensed or capitalized using GAAP. It is normally to the benefit of both tax-exempt and investor-owned hospitals to expense as many of the remodeling and renovation expenses as possible. This results in faster recovery of costs through reimbursement. Because of the time value of money, this results in reimbursement with greater purchasing power.

Miscellaneous Cost Items

Current regulations require hospitals to direct-apportion malpractice insurance. Medicare patients have historically been awarded fewer, as well as smaller, malpractice insurance settlements than have non-Medicare patients. This is due in part to the fact that the procedures that would have the greatest chance of resulting in a malpractice suit are performed less often on older patients and the fact that courts have awarded larger settlements to persons in their prime or childhood than they have to Medicare recipients. By requiring hospitals to direct-apportion malpractice insurance, less of this expense is allowed by the Medicare program.

Hospitals have for years been attempting to direct-apportion expenses. But the government has always disallowed direct apportionment of high Medicare expenses. Thus, the hospital industry is contesting in the courts the government's requirement to direct-apportion malpractice costs. It seems unlikely that a prudent judge will permit the government to allow direct apportionment of costs for others but not grant the same privilege to hospitals and other providers. Therefore, it is recommended that hospitals do not complete the malpractice apportionment schedule in the cost report. The intermediary will then require that the schedule be completed, but the hospital will have established its position. If the regulation is voided by the courts, the intermediary will be required to give the hospital credit automatically for any additional reimbursement. If, however, the hospital does not establish its position upon filing, the intermediary may not make the adjustment and may not allow the hospital to reopen its cost report to take advantage of its position.

To protect further the hospital's reimbursement, it is recommended that malpractice claims on Medicare recipients be disputed less vigorously than other malpractice claims. This will increase the hospital's Medicare malpractice experience. For most American hospitals, the additional reimbursement from Medicare will be substantially more than the cost of settling selected Medicare malpractice claims.

Charity care has been disallowed on the cost reports. The new law specifically excludes charity for cost reports, but the matter is still being disputed in the courts. Recently, courts have ruled that charity care is an allowable expense for Medicare. Thus, all hospitals should claim charity care on their cost reports. The preferred manner is to make charity care a deduction from total gross revenue by department. Another way to claim it is as an expense on the Medicare stepdown. In both cases, intermediaries at this writing are required to disallow the charity care. Thus, the hospital's inclusion of the charity care on the cost report is merely to establish its position. A claim for disputed items on the cost report guarantees that they will be allowed if the regulations change or the courts void applicable regulations.

Using the same logic, it is recommended that the hospital take all bad debts, credit card discounts, and other similar items. The preferred manner is to take these as expenses rather than as deductions from revenue. In this manner, the chances are greater that the costs will be allowed on Blue Cross cost reports, on other cost reports, in rate review hearings, and in other reporting.

The cost accounting techniques we have described are intended only to illustrate the type of thinking that should be used by reimbursement accountants. Most cost techniques are unique to the particular hospital or other institution. Financial personnel must constantly seek techniques that can be used in their institution to increase Medicare, Medicaid, and other cost reimbursement.

BLUE CROSS COST REPORTS

In approximately half of the states, Blue Cross plans reimburse hospitals according to a cost report rather than on a form of billed charges. Special care must be given to these Blue Cross cost reports.

As noted earlier, many Blue Cross cost reports ask the hospital to complete schedules or perform calculations that, by contract, the hospital is not required to do. Blue Cross often assumes a spillover from Medicare regulations onto their cost reports. This is logical and predictable. It is also logical and predictable that hospitals often assume a spillover of Medicare reimbursement principles to Blue Cross reports. This is especially true if the Blue Cross forms change to accommodate new Medicare regulations.

In this connection, it is important to remember that the Medicare and Medicaid cost reports do not necessarily follow GAAP. The reports are completed by following regulations promulgated by the Medicare Bureau, which is a part of HHS. Many of the Medicare rules, regulations, and other requirements are government budget-balancing devices. The hospital's contract for Medicare binds it to many of the Medicare regulations. But this does not mean that those regulations must be followed on other cost reports or for other rate-setting agencies.

If the Blue Cross contract does not specifically state that it binds the hospital to present and future Medicare regulations in the completion of the Blue Cross cost report, the hospital should assume that GAAP apply. The cost report forms are not binding. The Blue Cross contract is the instrument to which the hospital is bound. Therefore, extreme care is necessary when completing a Blue Cross cost report. This is especially true if the person completing the report is the same person who completes the Medicare cost reports. Care is also needed in the event that Blue Cross proposes a new contract or an addendum to an existing contract.

By the same logic, Medicare principles do not automatically apply to state rate-setting hearings or to cost contracts with nongovernment agencies. It is not uncommon for large corporations to have one set of financial statements for taxes, another for cost reporting, and a third for financial reporting. It should not be considered uncommon for a hospital to have one set of financial statements for cost reporting, a second for rate setting, and a third for financial reporting.

Chapter 5

The Cost Allocation Process

Medicare, Medicaid, and other cost payers pay only for the costs of revenue-producing patient care departments. To receive payment for housekeeping, administration, laundry, utilities, dietary, and other non-revenue-producing departments, the costs of these departments must be allocated to the revenue departments. This chapter examines some of the techniques that may be used to maximize reimbursement through cost allocations. (Current Medicare instructions and worksheets pertaining to the Medicare cost allocation process are contained in Appendix C. The process of completing the worksheets is commonly called the Medicare stepdown process. The Appendix C instructions and forms should be reviewed in conjunction with this chapter to gain a better understanding of the techniques discussed.)

OPTIONS

The majority of American hospitals and other providers have been guided simply by the forms themselves in the Medicare stepdown process. Most providers have failed to consider the other options that are available. Providers can change the sequence of allocations, can use alternative statistical bases, and can perform direct costing techniques to eliminate the need for allocations. In this section we examine each of these options.

Changing the Sequence of Allocations

To change the sequence of allocations, the provider must demonstrate a legitimate reason for the change and obtain approval from the intermediary. The reason should always be that the alternative sequence is more equitable. Thus, the provider should criticize the existing sequence as well as justify the proposed sequence. The request to the intermediary should include a reference to the following statement in the provider reimbursement manual:

> The cost of the non-revenue producing center serving the greatest number of other centers, while receiving benefits from the least number of centers, is apportioned first. Following the apportionment of the cost of the non-revenue producing center, that center will be considered closed and no further costs are apportioned to it.[1]

Many intermediaries will not allow any change in the sequence of allocating costs. However, if the hospital can prove that the change would produce a more accurate basis of allocation and that significant additional reimbursement will result, the requested change should be appealed. If the potential additional reimbursement is not significant, the proposed new sequence should be abandoned, but not before the intermediary has agreed to concede on another issue that is to the hospital's benefit. Any time that the hospital concedes one of its rights on a cost report issue, it should attempt to gain a benefit in another area of the cost report. Often, certain issues are challenged knowing they will be conceded. In these cases, the challenge merely serves to strengthen the hospital's position in negotiating another issue.

Using Alternative Statistical Bases

The statistical basis for allocating nonrevenue cost centers on the cost report is not optional. However, an alternative statistical basis may be used if the data for the existing basis are not available or it can be demonstrated that the proposed new basis will be a more accurate basis of allocation. The most common reason for using an alternative statistical basis is that information to use the recommended basis is not available. If a hospital wishes to change to new stepdown statistics, it is best to change its statistical reporting so that the previously used statistics are no longer available. The new statistics are then used. If the change is challenged in the audit process, the hospital accountant can say that the old statistics are not available so the best available alternative data were used.

Many hospitals continue to use existing allocation statistics because other recommended data were not available. If the recommended basis can now be obtained because of more sophisticated reporting systems, this alternative should be investigated. If the new data increase reimbursement, they should be used; if they do not increase reimbursement, they should not be used. If the new data significantly reduce reimbursement, the hospital should immediately discontinue gathering them. (Specific examples of alternative allocation bases are given in a later section.)

Using Direct Costing Techniques

Direct costing should always be referred to as expense identification or as another technique in correspondence or discussions with the intermediary. This is because direct costing has been used by many providers in recent years and may now have a negative psychological effect on some Medicare auditors.

Expense identification is a process of identifying the indirect expenses attributable to a cost center through accounting studies. Since the indirect expenses are known, there is no need to rely on statistical allocations to estimate the indirect expenses. This technique eliminates the need for cost allocation through the stepdown. If properly documented, direct expense identification can be shown to yield a significantly more accurate, as well as a more appropriate, allocation of costs. This fact makes it difficult for the intermediary to disallow the technique.

Opportunities to increase reimbursement through direct cost identification must be identified on an institutional basis. The specific examples identified in subsequent sections are not all-inclusive.

METHODS

The most common method of allocation is the single apportionment method, also called the stepdown method. This method recognizes that services rendered by certain nonrevenue-producing departments benefit other nonrevenue departments as well as revenue-producing cost centers. All of the costs of nonrevenue-producing departments are allocated to other departments according to available statistics. The costs are allocated only to the departments that follow in the cost allocation sequence. Once a department has been allocated to other departments, no other costs can be allocated to it; it is as if the department no longer exists. (Instructions and forms for using this technique are provided in Appendix C.)

The double apportionment method involves two separate and distinct stepdowns. In the first stepdown, costs are allocated to all departments, including those to which allocations have already been made. When a cost center has all of its costs allocated to other departments, it remains open to accumulate other allocated costs. At the completion of this first stepdown, most of the nonrevenue-producing departments have small amounts of money that have not been allocated. These small amounts represent allocations from other nonrevenue departments.

The second stepdown of a double apportionment is to allocate the relatively small amounts in the nonrevenue departments. This stepdown is performed exactly like the single stepdown apportionment, except that the departmental costs accumulated in the last column of the first stepdown are used rather than the department costs accumulated in the trial balance of expenses. In completing the second stepdown, departments are closed after their costs have been allocated. They do not receive additional allocations.

In practice, the double apportionment stepdown is seldom used on the Medicare cost report. Essentially, the results of a double apportionment are the same as those from a single stepdown. A double apportionment is thus not usually warranted. Most of the double apportionment stepdowns being used today are performed by a computer.

If permission is granted from the intermediary, a more sophisticated method of apportionment can be used. However, it is virtually impossible to perform an apportionment more sophisticated than double apportionment without the aid of a computer. And most approved computer programs do not utilize more sophisticated methods because they do not, in most instances, significantly change reimbursement. Thus, more sophisticated methods remain a seldom-used option. When they are used, they utilize either multiple apportionments or simultaneous equations.

PREPARING FOR APPORTIONMENT

Proper preparation is necessary in order to obtain maximum benefits from apportionment techniques. Such preparation includes timing, cost ranking, and consideration of limits and ceilings.

Timing

As with accounting techniques, it is important to perform the techniques of cost apportionment as soon as practicable. If reimbursement for a service is poor, the first consideration should be a corporate reorganization to remove the service from the institution's cost report. The second most effective technique is direct costing to remove the service from apportionment.

In studying statistics to maximize reimbursement, it is most beneficial to create new cost centers. And in shifting costs through statistical studies, it is normally more effective to influence the statistics that are used in the first departments to be apportioned. In apportionment, if there are two different techniques that can be used, the technique that influences costs first is normally the more effective.

Cost Ranking

The hospital can often influence the manner in which costs are allocated. Before performing studies to determine the allocation statistics, the analyst should know the percentage of each department's revenue that is cost reimbursed. If a dollar can be shifted from a department that is 50-percent cost reimbursed into a department that is 70-percent cost reimbursed, the hospital will receive an additional 20 cents in reimbursement.

The tool used to determine department cost ranking is a ranking schedule, as explained in Chapter 4. This schedule ranks departments according to the percentage of revenue that is cost reimbursed. For ancillary departments, the percentage that is cost reimbursed is determined according to the following ratio of charges:

$$\frac{\text{Cost reimbursed revenue}}{\text{Total gross revenue}} = \frac{\text{Department cost}}{\text{reimbursement percentage}}$$

For routine care, special care, and other room-and-board cost centers, the percentage that is cost reimbursed is determined according to the following ratio of charges:

$$\frac{\text{Cost reimbursed patient days}}{\text{Total patient days}} = \frac{\text{Department cost}}{\text{reimbursement percentage}}$$

Cost reimbursed days include Medicare patient days, Medicaid patient days, and other patient days that are reimbursed according to a cost report. A ratio with patient days is used because room-and-board cost centers are reimbursed on a per diem basis.

The reimbursement specialist refers to the ranking schedule throughout the statistic gathering and testing process. In the process, an attempt is made to skew the statistics toward the high cost reimbursed departments until costs in those departments reach a limit or ceiling.

Limits and Ceilings

There are several limits and ceilings in the Medicare and Medicaid programs, and it is expected that the government will use such limits and ceilings extensively in future budget-balancing efforts. The most common limits for Medicare have been (1) the lower of cost or charges and (2) routine service limits prior to 1982. After 1982, the routine service limits were replaced by two different case mix limits (discussed in Chapter 8). The most common limits for Medicaid are (1) the number of covered days and (2) a per diem limit on skilled-nursing and long-term care facilities. Most of the money that is lost because a hospital is over one of these limits is not recoverable. There are also certain limits on therapy services, drugs, and other selected costs.

Because money lost because of limits is seldom recovered, these limits must be carefully watched. If a reimbursement specialist believes that a reimbursement limit will be reached, money should be transferred out of the applicable cost center and into a cost center in which there is further opportunity for reimbursement. Fortunately, a hospital normally knows that it will reach a ceiling several years in advance. If the controller is tracking trends, the precise year as well as the amount can be predicted, while there is still time to correct the trend.

It is important to remember that limits represent that portion of the reimbursement maximization process that should be dealt with most aggressively. Statistical bases, as well as cost studies chosen for the stepdown, should be used in efforts to limit the amount of cost in an area that has a potential problem with a limit or ceiling.

STEPDOWN TECHNIQUES

Once the hospital has considered the potential for limits, has prepared a current ranking schedule, and is aware of the importance of timing, specific techniques to maximize reimbursement in the cost allocation process can be implemented effectively. Some intermediaries will not allow the use of these techniques. However, it should be remembered that the intermediary has a view that is different from that of the hospital. If pursued, many of these techniques, though originally rejected by the intermediary, may be allowed.

Allocation Bases

The measure of square feet is the recommended basis for allocating several cost centers. The regulations do not specify building gross square feet (BGSF) or building net square feet (BNSF). BGSF includes all of the square feet in each building. BNSF excludes the common areas, for example, hallways, restrooms, and housekeeping closets. Common areas can also include waiting rooms and lounges if it is determined that such inclusion is to the hospital's advantage. Normally BGSF puts more expenses in the routine care cost centers; BNSF puts more in the ancillary and special care cost centers. After an examination of the ranking schedule and the potential for exceeding routine cost limits, the hospital can decide which basis to use.

Expenses in the administrative and general (A & G) category are allocated according to accumulated costs. It is often advantageous to charge certain expenses directly to the departments in the accounting process rather than leave them in A & G. This leaves fewer expenses to be allocated on the stepdown. This is especially beneficial if the hospital has a professional office building, a long-term care unit, or other cost centers in which reimbursement is limited.

Also, it is often beneficial to allocate depreciation based on actual depreciation by department rather than on square feet. This is especially true if the ancillary departments are relatively higher cost reimbursed than routine care. Department depreciation based on actual depreciation places more costs in coronary care and intensive care than depreciation based on square feet. Normally, special care areas have expensive monitoring and other equipment but fewer square feet. It may be advantageous to use construction costs per square foot for building depreciation. The cost per square foot of radiology and surgery is significantly higher than it is for other areas. If these departments are high cost reimbursed, building depreciation can be weighted to take advantage of this. In all new construction, the hospital should ask the contractor or construction manager to provide cost per square foot by department. The hospital need use this information only if it is beneficial.

The recommended basis for allocating employee health and welfare is gross salaries. This cost center includes Social Security, worker's compensation, disability, unemployment taxes, and other benefits. Health insurance can almost always be charged directly to the various cost centers, or it can be part of the employee health and welfare cost center. Charging health insurance directly to the departments normally shifts costs out of the ancillaries into routine care. Other fringe benefits can also be analyzed and charged directly to the departments rather than be allocated on the stepdown worksheet.

Operation and maintenance of plant includes utilities. The recommended basis is square feet. If the hospital has a professional office building or other nonreimbursed area that includes a large amount of square feet but uses relatively few utilities, that area should be metered separately. The cost of installing additional meters for steam, electricity, gas, water, air conditioning ducts, and other utilities is often recovered in one year through additional reimbursement. Some hospitals use cubic feet rather than square feet to allocate utilities. Repairs can be allocated based on specific maintenance work orders rather than on square feet.

Dietary is often allocated on patient days rather than on meals served. Allocation by patient days places more expense in special care units (that is, intensive care and coronary care) than allocation by meals served because many patients in the special care units do not receive meals; they receive nourishment from intravenous feeding. If it is to the hospital's advantage to allocate dietary costs on the basis of patient days, the number of meals served by cost center should not be used.

Restricted gifts must be offset against costs of the cost center for which the restricted gift is used. If the hospital has a nonallowable cost center, it would be advantageous to solicit a restricted gift for that center. Because of the restricted gift offset, the nonallowable cost center will then receive fewer allocated costs in the stepdown. This leaves more costs to be allocated to allowable cost centers and increases reimbursement. The terms of a restricted grant also can specifically exclude the cost of services provided to patients not covered under Medicare.

In preparing for the stepdown, the hospital should distinguish as many cost centers as possible. This enables the reimbursement accountant to combine centers to the hospital's advantage or to leave them separate. It may be advantageous, for example, to combine the labor room and recovery room or the delivery room and surgery. Some hospitals make the social service function a part of A & G rather than a separate cost center. The square feet in the waiting room for the clinic and for the emergency room can be considered either as parts of those departments or as parts of A & G.

In deciding the basis for allocation, it should be noted that using gross patient revenue for allocation automatically weights the statistics heavily toward inpatients. This is normally advantageous to the hospital. Many hospitals have one or more support functions that are performed directly by personnel in the revenue-producing departments. Surgery may be cleaned by surgery personnel rather than by housekeeping because it is a sterile atmosphere. In many hospitals, the patient rooms are cleaned by personnel on the nursing department payroll rather than by housekeeping personnel. Sometimes repairs for the laboratory, operating rooms, or other areas are not performed by maintenance department personnel. In each of these examples, the allocation statistics can either exclude or include the applicable areas. If included, the areas are charged twice for the applicable service on the cost report. If the area is a high cost reimbursed department, it is to the hospital's advantage to charge the department twice for the service. Medicare principles do not follow GAAP. In most instances this departure from GAAP reduces reimbursement. This technique uses Medicare principles to the hospital's advantage.

Medical records time can often be weighted to account for the lowest salary of the clerks assigned to outpatient records. Central supply can be allocated on hours of service rather than on cost of supplies. If surgery is a high cost reimbursed department, this takes advantage of the time spent on sterile surgical packs and autoclaving. Laundry can be allocated on pieces of laundry rather than on pounds of laundry. A weighting factor can be determined to account for pieces of laundry that must be pressed or folded. Sterile laundry, such as surgical drapes, can be given a greater weight than nonsterile laundry.

Many low-cost computer aids are available to improve reimbursement through allocation statistics. The opportunities are limited only by the creativity of the reimbursement accountant. Sometimes a hospital accountant will change to a more sophisticated basis without evaluating the reimbursement impact, or the hospital will use a computer service merely because of the accuracy and sophistication it offers. Such moves should be avoided. The purpose for the use of reimbursement techniques should always be additional reimbursement. If the change does not produce more reimbursement, it should not be made, notwithstanding the sophistication it represents or the accuracy it offers.

An Alternate Method for A & G

For cost reporting periods ending on or after February 28, 1975, providers may elect to reclassify the A & G cost center into six component cost centers. (The regulations do not provide the alternative of reclassifying A & G into fewer than six components.) The required component cost centers, bases for allocation, and statistical allocations are as follows:

Component Center	Allocation Basis
1. Nonpatient telephones	1. Number of nonpatient telephone lines or number of instruments
2. Data processing	2. Machine time
3. Purchasing, receiving, and stores	3. Cost of supplies expensed
4. Admitting	4. Gross inpatient charges
5. Cashiering, accounts receivable, and collections	5. Gross charges
6. Other A & G	6. Accumulated costs

The intermediary can approve deviations from the above if the hospital can show that the deviation results in a more accurate allocation. The intermediary can also approve deviations if it is not possible to establish all six components with the provider's present accounting system.

For most free-standing, acute care hospitals, the approved method of breaking the A & G cost center into six separate components results in additional reimbursement. Once the election is approved, it is binding for the initially approved reporting period and all subsequent cost reporting periods. This alternative method requires additional work and record-keeping, and should not be elected if the projected benefits are small.

The intermediary will normally allow deviations from the statistical basis used and in the number of component cost centers established if the hospital does not have the necessary information to use the recommended methods. However, if reimbursement can be enhanced using other alternative bases, the hospital should not develop the statistics for reclassifying A & G as recommended. If available, the recommended information must be used, but there is no requirement to develop information that will have an adverse effect on the hospital's financial position.

Timing of Cost Studies

Cost studies to determine stepdown allocation statistics should be carefully planned. Laundry and linen cost is normally allocated to the different departments based on pounds of laundry used. The hospital should watch its in-house statistics carefully. When there is a relatively high percentage of cost-reimbursed patients, a pounds-of-laundry study should be performed. This skews the results toward the high Medicare departments, but it is still a valid study. A pounds-of-laundry study should not be conducted when the hospital has a high percentage of billed charge patients.

Dietary costs are often allocated to the cafeteria based on a weight-equivalent meals statistic. To develop this, the hospital chooses several average patient meals from the cafeteria menu and determines the cafeteria price. An average charge for a patient meal at cafeteria prices is determined. This average price is divided into gross cafeteria income to determine the number of equivalent cafeteria meals. The pricing for the cost study can be established either at a time when the cafeteria has relatively expensive menu items or at a time when the cafeteria has relatively inexpensive menu items. Breakfast is normally an inexpensive meal. If the hospital wants to maximize routine service costs and minimize the amount of cost allocated to the ancillaries, breakfast can be used several times in the cost study. If it is more beneficial to allocate expenses to the ancillaries, the more expensive afternoon meals can be used in the allocation study. Similarly, housekeeping assigned-hours-of-service studies can be performed during periods of inclement weather or periods of pleasant weather, during periods of high census or periods of low census.

The month of the year chosen to perform time studies for allocating nursing administration, nursing school, intern-resident service, and other schedules should be carefully determined. No study for cost allocation purposes should be performed without first determining the best time to perform the study. When the allocation of costs for an entire year is based on a small sample, there is an opportunity to obtain additional reimbursement by carefully choosing the time as well as the circumstances in which the study is performed.

MULTISERVICE DEPARTMENTS

Many hospitals have departments that serve hospital functions as well as nonhospital functions. These include medical schools, home health agencies, skilled nursing facilities, and nursing homes.

Partial Certification

If the hospital has a nursing home or skilled nursing facility, it is sometimes advantageous to certify only part of the facility. This technique has also been used successfully for free-standing nursing homes. Its merit lies in the fact that costs can be allocated more advantageously in a partially certified facility. The cost of caring for Medicare or Medicaid patients can be isolated, resulting in better reimbursement.

In using this technique, the expenses of the certified section must be isolated from the expenses of the noncertified section. This requires sophisticated accounting methods, as well as a record of time nursing personnel spend in each section. It also requires a cost finding system to allocate overhead costs separately to the certified section and the noncertified section. Also, the institution's chart of accounts must be expanded. However, if the additional recordkeeping is practicable, significant additional reimbursement is possible.

The Medicare regulations stipulate three requirements before a distinct part of a facility can be created:

1. The distinct part must be physically separate. The separate part can be a wing, a separate nursing station, or a separate floor. However, the certified beds do not have to be confined to a single part of the facility; they must only be distinctly separated from the noncertified beds.
2. The intermediary must be convinced that the hospital's accounting systems can furnish the information necessary to determine reasonable cost in the distinct part of the facility.

3. The provider must obtain permission from the state agency to certify only a portion of the facility. The request to do so must clearly describe the portion to be certified.

After the distinct part of the facility is established, the occupancy rate in the certified section cannot be more than 25 percent less than the occupancy in the noncertified section. If it falls below 25 percent, an adjustment must be made by the Medicare auditors to reallocate standby costs.

Medical School Hospitals

A hospital that is a distinct part of a medical school presents unique opportunities for reimbursement. Often many of its departments will serve the medical school as well as the teaching hospital. In such cases, the expenses of those departments must be allocated between these two functions before the hospital costs can be determined.

It is important to remember that, in such cases, costs can be allocated to the hospital for Medicare and other cost reports and also to the medical school for reports to the American Association of Medical Colleges, the state board of regents, and other entities. It is not immoral to claim costs more than once. As we have noted, large corporations may have one set of accounting records for income tax purposes, another set for marketing and pricing, and a third set for financial reporting. Similarly, teaching institutions can have one set of accounting records for cost reimbursement, another set for internal analysis, and a third set for reporting teaching costs. In each case, the analysis must start with a common trial balance of expenses, have a logical and defensible allocation, and reach a valid conclusion, depending upon the requirements. Often, cost accountants lose allowable reimbursement because they fail to claim valid hospital costs that were also claimed on medical school reports for a different purpose.

The allocation of costs between the medical school and the hospital should be completed on accounting worksheets rather than on the Medicare cost reports. If apportioned on the cost reports, the allocations become part of the Medicare process; if apportioned on worksheets, they become part of the accounting process of the institution. It is more difficult for the intermediary to challenge the internal accounting process than it is to challenge the Medicare reimbursement process. This is true for Medicaid, Blue Cross, and other cost payers, as well as for Medicare.

The allocation of costs between the medical school and the hospital can remain purposely vague. The auditors do not have a right to examine everything they request. The institution must prove only that the allocation is reasonable. Medicare does not have a right to substitute the intermediaries judgment for the judgment of the institution.

The statistics, cost studies, and other worksheets that are developed to support allocations between the medical school and the hospital should be voluminous. Medicare auditors do not understand medical schools. By making the records voluminous, a mystique is created that allows greater accounting flexibility.

Other Multipurpose Providers

A hospital that has a nursing home, home health agency, skilled nursing facility, or other separate provider should attempt to have a separate provider number for each function. This requires separate cost reports, but it also allows for greater flexibility in accounting. Often it is beneficial to have different intermediaries for each function. The Medicare program does not require that the intermediary for the hospital also be the intermediary for the skilled nursing facility, nursing home, or other separate function.

Medicaid limits and ceilings must be monitored closely. Normally, a high percentage of the nonhospital patients will be reimbursed by Medicaid, whose per diem limits, limitations on the number of covered days, and other regulations are more restrictive than Medicare regulations for hospitals. Therefore, it is usually to the institution's advantage to allocate as much overhead to the hospital as possible.

In a multipurpose provider setting, it is especially profitable to perform a corporate reorganization. This creates more opportunities to maximize reimbursement. Overhead cannot be apportioned to the functions of another legal entity, and overhead that is not apportioned away remains with the hospital and can be reimbursed on all of the hospital's cost reports.

NOTES

1. Reg. 405.453, Principle 2-3, paragraph d-1.

Chapter 6

Revenue and Pricing Strategies

REIMBURSEMENT FORMULAS

Medicare reimburses hospitals according to a ratio of program revenue to total gross revenue times allowable costs. Certain techniques can be used to increase the revenue portion of this reimbursement formula. The three reimbursement formulas that we will consider here are (1) the ratio of charges to charges applied to costs (RCCAC), (2) the cost-converter formula, and (3) the room-and-board formula. (Current Medicare regulations and forms relating to revenue and pricing strategy are contained in Appendix D. These should be reviewed in conjunction with this chapter to gain a better understanding of the techniques involved.)

The RCCAC Formula

The ratio of charges to charges applied to costs has been the basic formula used to reimburse hospitals since the beginning of the Medicare program. The RCCAC formula is calculated as follows:

$$\frac{MR}{TR} \times AC = HR$$

where: MR = Medicare gross revenue
TR = Total gross revenue
AC = Allowable costs
HC = Hospital reimbursement

The RCCAC formula assumes that if 50 percent of the department's gross revenue was for services to Medicare patients, then 50 percent of the cost of the department was incurred on behalf of Medicare patients. The formula assumes a direct correlation between charges and costs because all procedures are assumed to have the same markup.

Most Medicare regulations limit allowable costs. Relatively few regulations have been written to restrict reimbursement techniques that are used with the revenue half of the formula. At this writing, one of the most attractive opportunities for increasing reimbursement is with pricing strategy. There are very few regulations that restrict pricing techniques. The government has assumed that there is a basis for a logical, standard set of pricing practices in the hospital industry. This is a false assumption. In actuality, the hospital industry has not developed standard pricing practices for three major reasons:

1. The historical absence of a competitive environment: Hospital services have not been price sensitive.
2. The lack of financial sophistication in hospitals before the 1970s: Accounting was considered a necessary function, but it was not considered a crucial function until the advent of Medicare and the cost escalation and industry-government relationships of the 1970s.
3. The volume and diversity of the services offered: Labor intensive services pose difficult pricing problems. Given the diversity of the thousands of labor intensive services offered by hospitals, comparable pricing practices are a cost-prohibitive goal.

These three reasons have contributed to the opportunity to use pricing strategy in reimbursement maximization. In the more sophisticated hospitals, the traditional reasons for pricing are not considered significant; in such hospitals, prices are established primarily to increase cost reimbursement.

The Cost Converter Formula

Current Medicare worksheets (see Appendix D) use a cost converter formula rather than the RCCAC. The cost converter formula is mathematically derived from RCCAC as follows:

$$\frac{MR}{TR} \times AC =$$

$$\frac{MR \times AC}{TR} =$$

$$\frac{AC}{TR} \times MR$$

It should be clear that this is merely another way of stating the RCCAC formula. Therefore, in the present context, for purposes of understanding the principles and techniques of calculating reimbursement, we will continue to refer to RCCAC as the basic formula.

The Room-and-Board Formula

While the RCCAC formula is used to reimburse hospitals for all ancillary departments, a variation of the formula is used to reimburse hospitals for routine care, coronary care, intensive care, and other room-and-board cost centers. The room-and-board formula substitutes patient days for charges. Thus:

$$\frac{MD}{TD} \times AC = HR$$

where: MD = Medicare patient days
TD = Total patient days
AC = Allowable costs
HC = Hospital reimbursement

On the Medicare cost report, a per day allowable cost is calculated for each room-and-board cost center. This per diem amount is multiplied by the number of patient days to determine reimbursement. The formula assumes that if 50 percent of the patient days are Medicare patients, then 50 percent of the allowable cost should be attributed to Medicare. This assumes that all patient days require the same amount of expenses.

Many knowledgeable experts believe, as we do, that Medicare patients require significantly more nursing time and routine equipment than non-Medicare patients. However, this additional expense is difficult to quantify. For the period from July 1, 1969, through October 1, 1981, Medicare allowed an 8.5 percent routine nursing service differential as a reimbursable cost. This differential recognized the above-average cost of inpatient routine nursing care furnished to aged patients. The differential does not include inpatient days nor salaries for intensive care, coronary care, or other special care units. From October 1, 1981, through October 1, 1982, the allowed differential was reduced to 5.0 percent. Since October 1, 1982, no differential is recognized or allowed.

In calculating the differential, it is important to include all fringe benefits as well as all salaries of personnel assigned to the nursing units. The fringe benefits include payroll taxes, insurance benefits, employee discounts, and other benefits. Many of these benefits may be included in the general ledger expenses of the cost centers other than in routine nursing.

PRICING THEORY

Prices should always be established according to a comprehensive strategy. Since cost payers as well as bad-debt and charity care patients ignore the hospital's prices, pricing strategy becomes proportionately more effective as the percentage of patients who are cost reimbursed increases.

Room-and-Board Strategies

The room-and-board reimbursement formula utilizes a ratio of program days to total days rather than a ratio of program gross charges to total gross charges. Accordingly, the hospital cannot affect reimbursement through pricing. To increase reimbursement from room-and-board areas, the hospital must examine the patient classifications.

Private-room patient days are combined with semiprivate, ward, and other days. The hospital receives the same per diem reimbursement for all of these days. If a physician certifies that a private room is medically necessary, the hospital receives the same amount from Medicare but cannot charge the patient for the room differential. If a Medicare patient requests a private room but it is not medically necessary, the hospital can charge the patient for a room differential. The physician should be made aware of this and be encouraged to refuse to certify that a private room is medically necessary. Often, a physician will respond to the patient's request without knowing the financial consequences to the hospital. The hospital can receive additional reimbursement for isolation. If an isolation charge is established, the physician should be encouraged to request isolation, if feasible, rather than a private room.

As of October 1, 1982, the regulations impose a reduction in cost for what Medicare has termed a private-room subsidy. This does not change the basic reimbursement formula. As indicated in a later chapter, the reduction can be minimized by reducing the price spread between private and semiprivate room rates. The hospital must evaluate this to ensure that the additional reimbursement is not more than offset by a reduction in revenue from private pay and insurance patients.

The hospital receives additional reimbursement for coronary care, intensive care, and other special care units because the per diem costs are greater in special care units than in routine care units. The special care units—especially coronary care units—often have a higher percentage of Medicare than routine care costs. The government has established the following guidelines that must be followed to gain recognition of a special care unit:

- The unit must furnish services to critically ill patients. Such units include, but are not limited to, burn units, pulmonary care units, trauma units, psychiatric or neuro-intensive care units, and coronary care units.

- The unit must be in the hospital but be physically and identifiably separate from other units.
- There cannot be a concurrent sharing of nursing staff between special care units and less-intensive care units. However, two intensive care type units can share nursing staff.
- There must be specific written policies that include criteria for admission and discharge from the unit.
- At least one registered nurse must be present in the unit at all times.
- A minimum nurse-patient ratio of one nurse to two patients per day must be maintained. Included in this nurse-to-patient-day ratio are registered nurses, licensed practical or vocational nurses, and nursing assistants who provide patient care. Ward clerks, custodians, and other nonpatient care personnel do not count.
- The unit must have special life support equipment available for immediate use.

The potential for additional reimbursement is significant if the hospital can create additional special care units. In addition, special care patient days may increase the case mix for Section-223 limits. If a hospital is near its Section 223 limit for Medicare, the creation of special care units may be especially advantageous. Such a unit also significantly lowers the average cost of routine patient-day care by removing the more expensive patients from the average. This may be advantageous for Blue Cross cost reports or for rate-setting agencies. However, because the potential for additional reimbursement is significant, Medicare auditors often attempt to disallow the classification of a unit as a special care unit if the hospital does not have adequate documentation to prove it has complied with all of the requirements.

Ancillary Strategies for Increasing Medicare Revenue

Hospitals are reimbursed for ancillary departments according to the RCCAC formula, which uses a ratio of Medicare charges to total charges. The objective of pricing strategy is to accelerate the numerator of the ratio faster than the denominator. This results in a larger ratio applied to costs. The result is increased reimbursement.

To illustrate this principle, assume that the hospital has a department which (1) is 50-percent cost reimbursed, (2) has gross patient charges of $200,000, and (3) has total direct plus indirect allowable costs for Medicare of $150,000. The allowable costs for Medicare do not include bad debts, contractual allowances, or other expenses that are not recognized by Medicare. Reimbursement for this department is as follows:

$$\frac{\text{Medicare charges}}{\text{Total charges}} \times \frac{\text{Allowable}}{\text{costs}} = \frac{\text{Costs reimbursed}}{\text{by Medicare}}$$

or

$$\frac{\$100,000}{\$200,000} \times \$150,000 = \$75,000$$

Assume that there is a set of procedures in this department that is performed only on persons over 65 years of age. These procedures are virtually 100-percent Medicare. The hospital can increase gross revenue in this department by \$10,000 per year by raising the prices of the 100-percent Medicare procedures. The prices of all other procedures in the department remain unchanged. Reimbursement for this department will then change as follows:

$$\frac{\$110,000}{\$210,000} \times \$150,000 = \$78,571.43$$

Thus, cost reimbursement for this department has been increased by \$3,571.43 per year because of our pricing strategy.

To illustrate further, assume that, instead of raising the prices of Medicare procedures, the hospital raises the prices or procedures that are never performed for Medicare patients. This price increase adds \$10,000 to gross patient revenue for the year. The Medicare reimbursement according to the RCCAC formula will then be:

$$\frac{\$100,000}{\$210,000} \times \$150,000 = \$71,428.57$$

In this case, Medicare reimbursement has decreased \$3,571.43 because the hospital increased the prices only of non-Medicare tests.

These examples represent the situation in a typical hospital department. The \$10,000 price increase represents an opportunity to increase Medicare reimbursement by \$3,571.43, to reduce Medicare reimbursement by \$3,571.43, or to affect Medicare reimbursement throughout this \$7,142.86 range. If the hospital implements an across-the-board increase, all procedures in the department would receive a 5-percent price increase. There would be no effect on Medicare reimbursement because the numerator and denominator of the ratio would both increase by 5 percent.

The above principle is relatively simple to apply. The hospital can always increase Medicare reimbursement by raising the prices of those procedures that are more than 50-percent Medicare reimbursed more than the prices of those procedures that are less than 50-percent Medicare reimbursed. If a procedure is exactly 50-percent Medicare reimbursed, the prices have no effect on reimbursement.

Ancillary Pricing for Increasing Non-Medicare Revenue

It would not be prudent to consider only Medicare revenue when raising prices. A comprehensive strategy also considers the effect on billed charge revenue. In Chapter 2, the percentage increase gained from price increases was defined as 100 percent minus those classes of patients that ignore the hospital's prices. The formula was:

$$PI = 100 - (CR + BD + CC)$$

where: PI = Percentage increase in net revenue
CR = Percentage of revenue that is cost reimbursed
BD = Percentage of revenue that is bad debt
CC = Percentage of revenue that is charity care

This formula assumes an overall increase in which all procedures receive the same percentage price increase.

The formula to determine the price increase for billed charge reimbursement is:

$$BCI = BCP \times GRA$$

where: BCI = Net revenue increase from billed charge payers
BCP = Percentage of increase that is billed charge reimbursed
GRA = Gross revenue amount of price increase

In our example, we assumed that the department was 50-percent cost reimbursed and had gross patient charges of $200,000. Let us assume further that 10 percent of the revenue is bad debts and charity for the department. The department is thus 40-percent billed charge reimbursed.

In our first illustration, it was assumed that prices of 100-percent Medicare procedures were increased to raise gross revenue by $10,000 per year. The effect of this on billed charge payers is:

$$BCI = BCP \times GRA$$
$$BCI = 0 \times \$10,000$$
$$BCI = 0$$

The only gain to the hospital was the increased revenue from Medicare.

In our second illustration, we assumed that prices of 100-percent non-Medicare procedures were increased to raise gross revenue by $10,000 per year. The effect of this on billed charges payers is:

$$BCI = .80 \times \$10,000$$
$$BCI = \$8,000$$

Of the total increase, 20 percent can be attributed to bad debt and charity care patients. Although the hospital lost $3,571.43 in cost reimbursement, it gained an additional $8,000 from billed charge payers. If all procedures had received the same 5-percent increase, there would have been no effect on Medicare reimbursement, and the hospital would have received an additional $4,000. As this example illustrates, it is often advantageous to establish prices that reduce Medicare reimbursement but increase the total net income.

IMPLEMENTING PRICING

A comprehensive pricing strategy normally improves the net income of a hospital by 1.0 to 1.5 percent of gross patient revenue. If gross revenue is $10 million and the hospital has raised prices without considering the effect of cost reimbursement, there may be an opportunity to achieve $100,000 to $150,000 in additional net income. To achieve this additional net income, the hospital must first decide the overall price increase, then the departmental price increases, and finally the individual procedure price increases.

Overall Price Increase

In calculating the overall hospital price increase, the hospital must provide for working capital needs, prepare for eventual replacement of equipment and physical plant at inflated prices, keep up with appropriate technology, and provide for sound financial operations. It is important to remember that cost-based payers and bad-debt and charity-care patients are not affected by price increases. Prices must be increased enough to provide the required net gain solely from charge payers. It is thus necessary to recalculate contractual allowances each time a change is made in net gain or budgeted expenses.

Departmental Price Increases

To determine departmental price increases, the hospital must have a ranking schedule and a stepdown. The stepdown allocates nonrevenue-producing departments to the revenue-producing departments. This provides total revenue by department. The ranking schedule ranks departments according to the percentage of revenue that is cost reimbursed and the percentage of revenue that is billed charge reimbursed. This schedule ignores bad debt and charity.

When deciding the specific, overall average price increase to give each department, it is always more beneficial to give the largest price increases to the departments that have the highest percentage of billed charge reimbursement. The departments that have the highest percentage of cost reimbursed revenue should have the smallest markup on cost.

It is important in pricing strategy to consider all cost reimbursed revenue for a department. This includes Medicare, Medicaid, Blue Cross in half of the states, and many health maintenance organization (HMO) contracts. The high-cost reimbursed departments should always have a pricing structure that covers cost and also provides for some margin over cost. The hospital should never have a department that is priced to produce a projected loss.

Individual Procedure Price Increases

Individual procedure pricing is initiated after the overall increase for the department has been determined. It is a strategy that determines on a procedure-by-procedure basis what to charge for each test within the departments. This is a complex area in which pricing is difficult to implement. However, the potential for increased net income is substantial.

There are many computer programs available to maximize net revenue. All of the large certified public accounting firms either have a computer simulation model to assist their clients with pricing strategy or have access to a simulation model on a time-sharing basis. In addition, many consultants, shared-service data processing firms, and hospital associations have access to computer models to assist in pricing strategy. At this writing, however, most of the available simulation models do not have the ability to maximize reimbursement on a procedure-by-procedure basis. Most available programs only simulate departmentally. Yet, the advantages of procedure pricing are significant, and it is worthwhile to find a service that offers procedure-by-procedure capability.

To understand how procedure pricing affects net income, we will examine the extremes. Assume a department that (1) has total direct plus indirect costs for Medicare of $150,000 per year, (2) has present total gross revenue from all patients of $200,000, and (3) has a constant bad debt and charity care percentage of 10 percent. Table 6–1 illustrates net income for this department if it is 80-percent cost reimbursed, has 10-percent bad debt and charity, and is 10-percent billed charge reimbursed. In each case, we will raise net income by 5 percent, which is $10,000 per year.

As shown in the table, it is to the hospital's advantage to increase the prices of cost reimbursed procedures more than the prices of billed-charge reimbursed procedures in a high-cost reimbursed department. The reason

Table 6–1 High Medicare and Low Billed Charges Extreme

Charges:	Net Revenue
Before price increase:	
Medicare	$120,000
Billed charges	20,000
Total net income	$140,000
Raise only 100-percent Medicare procedures:	
Medicare	$121,429
Billed charges	20,000
Total net income	$141,429
Raise all procedures 5 percent:	
Medicare	$120,000
Billed charges	21,000
Total net income	$141,000
Raise only 100-percent billed charge procedures:	
Medicare	$114,286
Billed charges	25,000
Total net income	$139,286

is that raising the prices of billed charge procedures accelerates the denominator in the RCCAC ratio faster than the numerator. This produces less cost reimbursement. With only 10 percent of the revenue in the department as billed charges, the increase from these payers is less than the loss of Medicare revenue.

Table 6–2 illustrates net income for the department if it is 10-percent cost reimbursed, 10-percent bad debt and charity, and 80-percent billed charge reimbursed. The net revenue in all categories is significantly greater in Table 6–2 than in Table 6–1 because of the patient mix. With a greater percentage of billed charge patients, the hospital realizes more net income, notwithstanding the effect of pricing.

It should be noted that in a high-billed charges department, it is advantageous to raise the prices of non-Medicare procedures more than the prices of Medicare procedures. At this extreme, the RCCAC ratio is extraordinarily low and any increase in Medicare revenue is not enough to equal the additional income from raising prices of billed charge procedures. In our earlier example of a department that was 50-percent cost reimbursed, it was to the hospital's advantage to increase prices of billed charge procedures more than those of Medicare procedures.

Gains from pricing strategy are also affected by the markup between total costs and established rates for each department, by the percentage of revenue that is bad debt and charity care, by past pricing practices that

Table 6–2 Low Medicare and High Billed Charges Extreme

Charges:	Net Revenue
Before price increase:	
Medicare	$ 15,000
Billed charges	160,000
Total net income	$175,000
Raise only 100-percent Medicare procedures:	
Medicare	$ 21,429
Billed charges	160,000
Total net income	$181,429
Raise all procedures 5 percent:	
Medicare	$15,000
Billed charges	168,000
Total net income	$183,000
Raise only 100-percent billed charge procedures:	
Medicare	$ 14,286
Billed charges	168,889
Total net income	$183,175

established the present base, and by the formula by which non-Medicare cost payers reimburse the hospital. It is impossible to maximize pricing strategy gains fully without a computer simulation model. However, the hospital can use the following rules of thumb in establishing prices without the aid of a computer:

- If the department is high cost reimbursed, the prices of cost reimbursed tests should be kept relatively high.
- If a department is high billed charge reimbursed, the prices of billed charge tests should be kept relatively high.
- If there is a balance between billed charge reimbursement and cost reimbursement, the billed charge tests should be kept relatively high.

It should be noted that the gains from the use of these pricing strategies are relatively small when expressed as a percentage of total net revenue. Large gains either would not be approved in the hospital's rate review or would indicate that the hospital has arbitrarily set prices in a fraudulent manner. This does not mean that hospitals should ignore pricing strategy. A one percent gain in net revenue for a hospital that has $10 million in gross patient revenue is $100,000.

MEDICARE LOGS

Detailed logs are kept for Medicare, for Medicaid, and sometimes for Blue Cross and other cost payers. The following principles relating to Medicare logs are also applicable to other cost payer logs.

The Need for Logs

Medicare logs are records of the information and details from the billing forms. They are maintained solely for Medicare purposes. The log summaries are used on the cost reports.

The intermediary also keeps logs of covered services and days. If the hospital does not maintain accurate Medicare logs, the intermediary data must be used. If there is a discrepancy between the hospital data and the intermediary data, it must be reconciled or the intermediary data will be assumed to be correct.

Medicare logs provide several advantages to the hospital, in addition to providing a cross-check on the intermediary data. In keeping a Medicare log, the hospital must compare the patient bill with the remittance advice that is received with the check from the intermediary. This reconciliation alerts the hospital to amounts that have been disallowed. Often, amounts that should have been covered are disallowed. In these cases, the hospital can take immediate action. At other times, amounts are disallowed because they should have been paid by the patient as a coinsurance amount or patient deductible. Reconciliation of the remittance advice with the bill is the only way to learn when a supplemental bill should be sent to the patient. If logs are not maintained, such situations could result in lost revenue.

Probably the most valuable benefit to be gained from keeping Medicare logs is the ability to know when Medicare has lost a bill or made an input error in its data processing system. The log enables the hospital to make a timely delineation of unpaid claims. As part of the monthly closing procedures, the hospital can review unpaid claims and follow up if payment has not been made.

Though the ability to recover lost income is probably the greatest benefit to be gained from Medicare logs, the assurance of reimbursement on a more timely basis is another advantage. At year end, the intermediary logs are created from the remittance advices; these represent only paid claims. However, the amount of claims that have been billed but not paid may be significant. Without the hospital's logs, the billed but unpaid claims would be included in the following year's settlement. But hospitals are faced with cash shortages as well as inflation, and receiving reimbursement in the current year rather than in the subsequent year is an important advantage. Also, if revenue from the current year is combined with that of the following year, reimbursement from the RCCAC formula is reduced. This is because of year-end price increases. By having revenue at the previous year's prices in the formula, the ratio is reduced inappropriately, resulting in less reimbursement.

A final advantage of Medicare logs is in the information they provide on billing requirements. Medicare requirements for billing change constantly. The exercise of reconciling the remittance advice with the bills and the required follow-up alerts the hospital to these changes on a timely basis.

Some hospitals do not maintain Medicare logs. Instead, they use the intermediary data at year end to file their cost reports. These hospitals are at the mercy of the intermediary's figures. This practice does not result in total allowable reimbursement because there is no opportunity to find lost claims, to challenge disallowed amounts, or to reconcile the timing of payments. The importance of proper maintenance and accuracy of Medicare logs cannot be overemphasized.

Log Format

If manual entries are used, the Medicare logs should be maintained on columnar accounting sheets with the patient claims in the vertical format and the data pertaining to each claim on the horizontal format. Most Medicare logs are kept either totally or partially on a manual basis. The data pertaining to each claim, shown in Exhibit 6–1, are normally kept on 40-column pads. Each page is totaled; and, either monthly or quarterly, the page totals are summarized.

A separate log is kept for inpatient and for outpatient departments. The outpatient logs are similar to the inpatient logs except that fewer columns

---

Exhibit 6–1 Inpatient Medicare Log Data

1. Patient name	12. Total room and board
2. Health insurance number	13. Total ancillaries
3. Date of admission	14. Noncovered amounts
4. Date of discharge	15. Deductibles/coinsurance
5. Date benefits are exhausted	16. Date billed
6. Lifetime reserve days	17. Date paid
7. Leave days	18. Deductions
8. Covered days	19. Amount paid
9. Part-B coverage	20. Remittance advice number
10. Column for each ancillary	21. Column for Part-B ancillary amounts
11. Column for each level of covered days	

are required because less information is required on the Medicare outpatient billing form.

Posting the Logs

Medicare logs are posted at the time of billing to the intermediary. When the remittance advice is received from the intermediary, all of the detail is compared to the information on the log. Discrepancies are then investigated and resolved.

Adjustments to the bill are often required because of late charges, denials of service, unmet coinsurance or deductibles, or for other reasons. There are three ways to enter adjustments on the log:

1. Post the adjustments on the next available line of the log.
2. Post the adjustments on a separate adjustments log, leaving the original log unchanged.
3. Post a debit line that eliminates the original entry, and reenter a credit line stating the corrected amount of the billing.

On inpatient revenue, the logs should always be posted from the bill. Adjustments are posted after the remittance advice is compared to the bill. Inpatient coverage should have been verified. Therefore, there will be few required adjustments. On outpatient logs, there are normally numerous adjustments. This may be because the outpatient deductible has not been met, because the patient is not covered under Part B, or for other reasons. Because of the numerous adjustments, some hospitals have elected to post the outpatient logs from the remittance advices rather than from the bills. This is acceptable only if the hospital matches the claims to the remittance advice before posting to the log.

Periodically, the hospital's per diem rate or discount rate is adjusted. When this is done, the total amount of retroactive adjustment should be posted on one line of the log. It is not necessary to adjust each patient claim individually.

Posting revenue logs is extremely tedious and boring to most people. Even if the logs are computerized, the reconciliation to the remittance advice and the posting of adjustments are often done manually. Yet, although the work is time-consuming and detailed, the benefits are substantial.

ACCOUNTING TECHNIQUES

Hospitals often give discounts to certain classes of patients or have separate charge structures for some revenue sources. Dual pricing is normally initiated in order to remain competitive or to offer a service to the medical staff. Referred laboratory tests, in which hospitals process lab tests or specimens obtained from physicians' offices, are common examples.

Medicare regulations require that all classes of patients "receive the same markup." Without supporting documentation, the intermediary will interpret this to mean that all classes of patients "will be charged the same price." On the cost report, the intermediary will gross up the revenue for the discounted procedures to equal the gross revenue without a discount. This increases the denominator of the RCCAC ratio but leaves the numerator unchanged. In this way, significant Medicare reimbursement may be lost.

If the lower price can be cost-justified, the lower priced procedures do not have to be grossed up. In our example, the hospital can document the fact that the cost to process lab tests for patients seen in a physician's office is substantially less than the cost to process identical lab tests for hospital patients. The savings in this case result from, among other things, the fact that:

- There is no sample collection cost for referred lab tests.
- Samples from physician offices can be batched for processing.
- If the physicians rather than the patients are billed, there are fewer billing collection and cashiering costs and bad debts.
- Medical records requirements and other patient regulations are not all applicable to tests performed for physicians.
- Samples from physician offices can be processed during slack hours; no overhead or other salary premiums should be affected.

Once the hospital has determined the cost of processing both classes of samples, the same markup is applied to both to arrive at charges acceptable to Medicare.

Intermediaries as well as regional Medicare offices are reluctant to allow dual pricing. However, the Medicare regulations are clear: If two price structures can be cost-justified, no grossing up is required; if two price structures can be partially cost-justified, the lower-priced charges must be grossed up only for that portion of the discount that was not justified. It is often advantageous to hire Medicare specialists from accounting firms or consulting firms to develop the necessary documentation to support a dual-pricing situation.

Interim Payments

Hospitals are reimbursed for Part-A inpatient hospital services either as a percentage of billed charges or as an average cost per diem based on estimated reasonable costs. For outpatient and Part-B inpatient costs, the hospital interim rate is a percentage of billed charges. Interim-rate calculations based on a percentage of billed charges are more common than those based on per diem amounts for Part-A inpatients. For most hospital accounting systems, an interim-rate calculation based on a percentage of billed charges is easier to complete.

The intermediary reviews the interim rate amount periodically to determine whether an adjustment should be made. The hospital should insist that any interim-rate determination include a calculation for inflation. If beneficial to the hospital, the interim-rate review should also be seasonally adjusted.

The Medicare regulations permit a hospital to receive periodic interim payments (PIP) rather than a percentage of current billings. There are specific requirements that must be met before a hospital qualifies for PIP. However, the requirements are easy to meet and almost any American hospital can qualify. The intermediary must approve the request for PIP, but this approval is seldom withheld.

Under PIP, the hospital receives from Medicare a predetermined amount every two weeks. The amount is the same regardless of the patient census. The amount is calculated by the intermediary, using the following formula:

$$\frac{(C - B) \times D}{PI} = PIP$$

where: C = Estimated cost per inpatient day
B = Estimated beneficiary bad debt and coinsurance amounts per inpatient day
D = Projected annual Medicare days
PI = Payment interval factor

The payment interval factor is normally 26, because most PIP payments are made biweekly. The hospital can request that the payment interval be longer than two weeks but not longer than once per month. The hospital can also request that seasonal variations be considered in calculating PIP payments.

PIP is most beneficial to those hospitals that are experiencing a long collection-time lag for Medicare claims. If, on the average, a hospital is paid by the intermediary for Medicare claims within two weeks after the patient is discharged, the only benefit from choosing PIP is the ability to predict cash flow with more certainty. If the collection time lag between patient discharge and receipt of payment from Medicare averages more than two weeks, the hospital should request PIP.

With PIP, the hospital accounting becomes more complex. In addition, there are additional recordkeeping and reporting requirements. Because of the additional recordkeeping, as well as the relatively short Medicare collection-time lag in most regions, most American hospitals have not chosen PIP.

Other Considerations

Bad debts, collection agency fees, charity care, credit card discounts, and other revenue offsets should, whenever possible, be classified as expenses rather than as deductions from revenue. Collection agency fees are an allowable administrative expense for Medicare but would not be reimbursed as a deduction from revenue. Most other revenue offsets are treated as revenue deductions for the Medicare cost report. However, as expenses, they may be allowed on Blue Cross and other cost reports. This inflates the hospital's expense base. However, this may be a significant advantage if proposed hospital controls are mandated by the federal or state governments.

Other accounting techniques that can be used to the hospital's advantage apply to negotiations with physicians on hospital contracts. (This subject is discussed in detail in a subsequent chapter.) The techniques involve having as much as possible of the physicians' payments classified as Part-A administrative. The physicians' administrative functions should be delineated in the actual contract. If the hospital has combined billing for professional and hospital charges for selected ancillaries, the contract should state whether bad debts will be separated or treated as a percentage of billing.

Finally, it should be noted that revenue from Medicare and other cost payers has been significantly increased by many institutions through corporate reorganizations. This technique is discussed in a subsequent chapter.

Chapter 7

The Apportionment Process

In using techniques to determine which costs are apportioned to Medicare, the reimbursement specialist must be on firm ground, since such costs are difficult to adjust after the report is filed. In this connection, it is important to remember that prudence and common sense are not principles of reimbursement. The penalizing practices of Medicare have made what would normally be considered prudent business decisions imprudent as well as costly. (Current Medicare instructions and forms pertaining to the apportionment process are contained in Appendix E. These should be reviewed in conjunction with this chapter to gain a better understanding of the techniques discussed.)

ACCOUNTING PRINCIPLES

Manuals, Letters, and Pronouncements

Many of the principles governing apportionment are the result of HHS regulations, by which hospitals and other providers are bound. Others are contained in HCFA manuals, intermediary letters, provider letters, rulings, and general policies. Providers are not bound by the latter principles; only the intermediary is bound by them. Yet, intermediary auditors often do not distinguish between regulations and other pronouncements, because for them there is no difference. This is an important point to remember when an intermediary disallows a technique or a direct cost study.

The regulations require that hospitals maintain comprehensive, as well as auditable, statistical and accounting records. The apportionment of expenses to Medicare, Medicaid, and other cost-based programs is based on measures of service derived from statistical and accounting records. Most of these apportionments are based on averages. Whenever a deviation from the averages would result in additional reimbursement, there is a potential opportunity to increase reimbursement. However, the deviation must normally be accomplished in the accounting system. If there is not a uniform level of services being received by all classes of patients for a given service, the hospital must provide for this in its accounting records.

Basis for Apportionment

Ancillary services are apportioned to the different programs based on a ratio of charges. The hospital must, therefore, maintain adequate records of charges by program. There are two general rules governing ancillary revenue that is ultimately used to apportion expenses: (1) The charges must be uniformly applied to all classes of patients, and (2) the charges for services must be consistently related to the cost of providing those services.

Uniform Application

In order to maximize reimbursement under the first rule, the hospital must carefully examine its classification of patients. Many hospitals perform laboratory tests for patients of physicians on the medical staff. In order to remain competitive with independent outside laboratories or to provide an incentive for the medical staff to use the hospital, discounts are often required on referred laboratory tests. If the hospital offers discounts to a class of patients, the charges must be grossed up for Medicare purposes. This is a requirement that significantly reduces reimbursement. To illustrate this, assume the following:

- The hospital laboratories have $50,000 in Medicare revenue.
- The laboratories have $100,000 in gross patient revenue for hospital patients and $20,000 of revenue from tests performed on samples sent from physician offices. This $20,000 would be $40,000 if the full hospital rate were charged.
- Direct plus indirect cost for the laboratories on the Medicare cost report is $150,000.

If the discount to the referred laboratory samples is not grossed up, Medicare reimbursement for the laboratories is as follows:

$$\frac{\$50,000}{\$120,000} \times \$150,000 = \$62,500$$

If the revenue from referred specimens is grossed up to the normal hospital charges, the reimbursement is as follows:

$$\frac{\$50,000}{\$140,000} \times \$150,000 = \$53,571$$

In this example, the hospital receives $8,929 less in reimbursement, and there is no possible way to recover this. Therefore, it is beneficial to structure the accounting system to exclude these patients. If they are the physician's patients and not the hospital's, the revenue is classified as other operating income. As another operating revenue, the charges are not grossed up. The expenses for the services are apportioned through direct costing techniques or as a revenue offset on Schedule A–8. By not classifying referred lab tests as being performed for hospital patients, reimbursement is usually greater. This technique can also be used in other ancillary departments. For the technique to be most effective, the hospital should bill the physician and not the patient. If this is not possible, then the hospital should have a written agreement that states that the hospital will bill the "physician's" patients on behalf of the physician. The agreement can state that the charge to the physician will be equal to the amount collected.

Many hospitals are multipurpose providers. In addition to acute care patients, they may have a skilled nursing facility or other type of nonambulatory patient care facility. It is sometimes better to account for ancillary tests performed for the patients in such facilities as outpatient revenue rather than as inpatient hospital revenue.

If inpatients of another facility are transported to the hospital for treatment, the accounting records and billing system can be set up to record the applicable revenue as patient income or as other operating income. This is another example of a potential for additional reimbursement through classification of patient income. Thus, a review should be made of all services being provided and of the classification of the resulting revenue.

Charges Consistent with Cost

The second rule requires that charges be consistently related to the cost of providing service. The health care industry does not have uniform, generally accepted, cost accounting practices and pricing structures. The regulations do not require that all classes of patients be charged the same amount; they require that any dual-pricing structure must be cost-justified. That is, all classes of patients must receive the same markup on costs.

If the hospital processes laboratory specimens for the staff physicians, there is often a discount given. The hospital should cost out the processing of inpatient tests and the cost of tests processed for physicians. If each group of tests is given the same markup, Medicare regulations are satisfied.

If the hospital can cost-justify part of a discount given to a class of patients, it will be required to gross up charges only from the point at which the discount was cost-justified.

Applicable cost savings that have been identified by hospitals include those for specimen collection, the processing of referred specimens in large batches, no-stat tests for referred tests, and lower overhead. The savings involved must be documented; indeed the hospital should be prepared to provide a considerable amount of documentation to satisfy Medicare regulations.

Cost-justifying all or part of a dual-pricing situation is thus tedious and time-consuming. The Medicare Bureau may ask for what appears to be excessive documentation. However, the resulting increased reimbursement is normally substantial.

Malpractice Costs

Effective for cost reporting periods beginning after June 30, 1979, the Medicare cost report includes forms to direct-apportion malpractice insurance. The rules require that the cost of malpractice premiums and self-insurance fund contributions be accumulated separately and directly apportioned to Medicare, based on a five-year average of losses paid to Medicare patients divided by total losses paid. If the hospital does not have any malpractice loss experience, it must use the government averages.

Many hospitals are settling small Medicare malpractice claims more readily than others in order to skew the Medicare loss experience upward. This is a prudent financial management principle that has been successfully used in other situations for many years. Accountants are taught to evaluate the cost-benefit ratio of expenditures. If the benefits through the reimbursement process of settling a Medicare malpractice claim without protest are greater than the amount of the settlement, the hospital should pay the claim.

Many hospitals do not complete the malpractice apportionment schedule when they file the cost report. The omission is disclosed in the cover letter in order to avoid any fraud and abuse penalty. It is believed that the courts will eventually eliminate the requirement that malpractice insurance be apportioned directly. In that case, if the hospital has not completed this form, the intermediary will adjust prior year reports to remove adverse audit adjustments.

On any apportionment form that may be required in the future, the hospital should look for ways in which the form can be influenced through the accounting system. It should then determine whether to complete the form. By following these two steps, reimbursement is increased, regardless of the outcome.

If the hospital is self-insured for medical malpractice, a malpractice reserve fund must be maintained. The money in this fund is invested. The hospital should obtain a separate 501(C)(3), tax-exempt ruling from the IRS for this fund. The self-insurance reserve is managed by a trustee and does not automatically qualify as tax-exempt under the hospital tax exemption. The additional exemption for the insurance reserve fund is not difficult to obtain.

HOSPITAL-BASED PHYSICIANS

There are numerous opportunities to increase reimbursement from fees paid to hospital-based physicians. Often this can be accomplished without changing the amount of money paid to the physicians.

Part-A Costs

The Medicare manual defines provider-based physicians as those physicians who perform services in a provider setting and have a financial arrangement under which they are compensated by or through an extended care facility, home health agency, clinic, hospital, rehabilitation agency, or public health agency. There are four different categories of service that a physician can perform for a hospital:

1. administrative (Part A)
2. teaching (Part A)
3. clinical (Part B)
4. ancillary department (Part B)

It is very difficult to distinguish between payments to physicians for professional services that are Part A and payments to physicians for professional services that are Part B. Part-A (administration and teaching) services are reimbursable costs. Part-B (patient care) services are reimbursed to either the hospital or the physician, based on billing screens established by Medicare. Part-B costs are not necessarily affected by increases in amounts paid by Part A. Therefore, it is normally to the hospital's advantage to identify as much Part-A cost as possible.

The hospital should have a contract with the physician to provide management for the physician's department. This includes hiring, evaluating, and discharging employees. It also includes preparing budgets, monitoring, attending meetings, scheduling, ordering, inventorying supplies, and handling other duties required by management. In many cases, the physician will delegate these functions to a nonphysician manager. However, if the contract defines the functions as part of the physician's responsibility, a portion of the remuneration paid can be allocated to Part A.

In addition to stipulating administrative duties, the contract can require the physician to be responsible for professional administration. This includes adherence to accreditation requirements, quality control, and evaluation of technicians. The contract should further state that the physician represents the department at meetings of the medical staff and on appropriate committees. The pathologist's contract can require the physician to perform autopsies. All of these functions are performed by the physician regardless of how the contract reads. However, by making them part of the contract, additional costs can be allocated to Part A.

Many hospitals have technology schools, nursing programs, employee orientations, and other educational efforts. If the physician is involved in any of these, it should be delineated in the contract so that Part-A costs can be allocated to teaching. If the hospital participates in a teaching program of another institution, such as a licensed practical nursing program or resident program, the provider-based physicians normally assist in teaching the students. If this is a requirement of their contracts, Part-A costs for the function can be allocated on the hospital cost report.

Emergency-room physicians are normally responsible for some administrative functions. This is especially true for emergency room physicians who are on duty at night and on weekends. If such functions are made a part of their contracts, some Part-A costs can be allocated to them. The physicians who read electrocardiograms or electroencephalograms normally provide supervision over the technicians and are responsible for the quality of the procedures. In other instances, physicians are responsible for employee health services. Indeed, all physicians who are paid by the hospital provide some service that can be related to Part-A costs. Hospitals should define all such services and determine specific compensation rates for them.

Percentage Agreements

In many hospital departments, physicians are compensated on a percentage of gross patient revenue. If a hospital raises its prices in these departments, the physicians automatically receive a percentage of the departments, the physicians automatically receive a percentage of the price increase. The major disadvantage of this type of arrangement is that the price increases are diluted. A major advantage, however, is that the physicians who receive a percentage of revenue will often educate other members of the medical staff on the benefits of ordering more diagnostic tests. Another advantage is that there are normally fewer lost charges if the physician who is the head of the department receives a percentage of revenue. Both of these advantages result in increased total gross revenue.

It is preferable to have percentage contracts defined as a percentage of net patient revenue rather than gross patient revenue. In this manner, if bad debts, charity, discounts, and contractual allowances increase, the physician shares in the reduction of revenue.

Moonlighting Residents

Most residents are fully licensed physicians who are training in a specialty. If the services of residents are not within the scope of their training program, their hospital compensation is treated exactly as if they were not residents. Residents who moonlight in the emergency room of a hospital should not be considered residents in a nonapproved teaching program. If they are so considered, the applicable costs are needlessly excluded on the cost report. This is a common error on Medicare cost reports.

APPORTIONMENT TECHNIQUES

Direct Apportionment

Many expenses can appropriately be apportioned to applicable departments or areas. This should be accomplished through the general ledger system, if practicable. An example of this technique is in the apportionment of housekeeping and maintenance costs for a professional office building. Housekeeping and maintenance cost per gross square foot is less in an office building than in a hospital. Since professional office buildings are not an allowable cost for Medicare, it is to the hospital's advantage to allocate as little cost as possible to this area.

A restricted gift to a nonreimbursable cost center, such as a professional office building, increases Medicare reimbursement. Restricted gifts are offset against expenses before the stepdown to allocate indirect costs. Administrative and general overhead is allocated on accumulated costs. If a nonreimbursable cost center's expenses are reduced, it will result in less overhead being allocated to that area.

A gift that is restricted to a particular overhead function of a nonreimbursable cost center can also increase reimbursement. If the hospital accepts a gift that is to be used for maintenance and housekeeping in a professional office building or other nonreimbursable cost center, no maintenance or housekeeping expenses are allocated to this area on the stepdown. Overhead that is allocated to a nonreimbursable cost center is not available to be allocated to patient care cost centers.

Pharmacy and central supply distribution should be examined to determine whether there is a potential for increased reimbursement. In some hospitals, aspirins, small bandages, and other nonpatient charge items are not charged to the various hospital departments. They remain in pharmacy and central supply to be apportioned on the stepdown. It may be cost effective to charge these items directly to the user departments.

Outside consulting is often charged to administrative and general. If the consulting is primarily for a patient care department, however, it is often beneficial to charge it directly to the department receiving the benefit. Interest expense can often be charged directly to the department to increase reimbursement. For example, if funds are borrowed to purchase x-ray equipment, the interest expense can be charged directly to radiology. The intermediary may challenge direct apportionment of interest expense. However, the fact that a treatment of an expense on the general ledger is challenged does not necessarily make it improper.

Revenue Offsets

GAAP define bad debt expense as an appropriate cost of doing business. Hill-Burton charity care is also an appropriate expense. However, the Medicare manual does not allow a hospital to take bad debts or charity as an allowable expense.

Nevertheless, hospitals should take both bad debts and charity as expenses on cost reports. To comply with the fraud and abuse act, this must be disclosed when filing the report. Such revenue offsets will be contested in the courts for many years; if the hospital has taken these on the cost reports, it has protected its right to appeal any adverse audit adjustments made by the intermediary. This right can be exercised if the court system decides to allow such expenses for Medicare.

Many Blue Cross cost reports allow bad debts as an allowable expense, notwithstanding the fact that Medicare does not. Unless specifically excluded, bad debt is also allowed as an expense for rate-setting agencies. In general, bad-debt expense is more beneficial to the hospital than charity-care expense.

The difference between charity care and bad debts is primarily a matter of judgment at the discretion of the hospital. Charity care should, therefore, be closely monitored. The optimal amount of charity care is the exact amount necessary to fulfill the Hill-Burton obligation, which is either (1) three percent of the operating budget of the facility less Medicare and Medicaid, or (2) ten percent of the federal construction aid originally received. After the lower of these two options has been met, an attempt should be made to classify all remaining nonpaid care as bad debt. If this is closely monitored, the hospital can set its charity criteria in a manner that produces the required amount of charity care without adjusting its standards during the year.

Subsidies

Many hospitals receive subsidies. The subsidy may be from a medical school, a county, a state, a municipal government, or from some other entity. In such cases, it is important to have unrestricted or nondirected subsidies. For example, if a hospital receives a county subsidy for ambulance service, it is normally to the hospital's benefit to ask for an undirected or unrestricted subsidy. The hospital can still agree to provide ambulance service for the county but will not have to offset the subsidy against costs.

This same principle applies to other subsidies. If a medical school gives a teaching hospital a subsidy to improve the operations of a particular department, that subsidy is offset against costs of that department for Medicare. It is far better to receive nondesignated funds and agree separately to provide the desired service.

If the hospital receives a grant, it should request that the grant document specify that this is a seed-money grant. Seed-money grant revenue is not offset against costs for Medicare. Operating grants must be offset against costs. Most agencies will agree to put the term *seed money* in the grant document if the reasons for this request are made clear to them.

Related Organization Costs

Costs from a related organization should be apportioned to the hospital. This includes interest, janitorial, maintenance, repair, and other costs. An apportionment of indirect overhead costs should be made for functions of county, state, home office, and other related organizations. The costs, including overhead, are then apportioned to the hospital from the related organizations.

Sometimes a government or other related organization will borrow money for a purpose not related to the hospital and give the hospital a subsidy from nonborrowed funds. For example, a county may give the hospital a subsidy that is paid out of general fund tax revenues and then borrow money to purchase equipment for the school system or for some other purpose. If politically feasible, it is better for the county to pay for the school system equipment and to borrow money to pay the hospital subsidy. If money is borrowed for payment to the hospital, a significant portion of the interest expense is reimbursed through the cost reports. Additional money is thereby paid into the county.

Often, a county will give a hospital a subsidy to offset the loss on ambulance service. As stated earlier, this subsidy is offset against the cost of running the ambulance service. It would be better if the hospital agreed to run the ambulance service for the county and, in a separate agreement, the county agreed to pay a nondirected subsidy to the hospital. The nondirected subsidy is not offset against costs on the Medicare or Medicaid cost reports.

Labor Room Days

The Medicare manual requires that persons in the labor room be counted as part of the midnight census, notwithstanding the fact that no beds have been assigned to the expectant mothers and no routine care charge is made. The hospital industry is opposing this regulation through the courts. Until the matter is totally settled by the courts, hospitals should not include labor room days in total day care. To do so lowers the Medicare per diem. Since Medicare recipients do not use the labor room, the inclusion of labor-room days does not add allowable days to the calculation. The effect is to reduce reimbursement.

To illustrate this, assume that a hospital has 1,000 labor room days, 10,000 Medicare routine care days, 20,000 total routine care days, and $3,000,000 of cost for routine care on the cost report. If labor room days are not included, the reimbursement for routine care would be:

$$\frac{\$3,000,000}{20,000} \times 10,000 = \$1,500,000$$

If labor room days are included, the reimbursement for routine care would be:

$$\frac{\$3,000,000}{21,000} \times 10,000 = \$1,428,571$$

By including the 1,000 labor room days, the hospital has lost $71,429 in reimbursement.

If a hospital follows Medicare instructions to include labor room days and the courts rule in favor of the providers, that hospital will be able to exclude such days from all future cost reports. However, it will have lost the right to do so on all previous cost reports. If a hospital has excluded labor room days and the intermediary has made an audit adjustment to include them, the hospital is in a better position. In this instance, if a court rules in favor of the providers, the intermediary will have to amend prior year cost reports to reverse its audit adjustment. In short, on any issue being contested in the courts, the hospital should, in completing the cost report, assume the issue has been won. The intermediary will make an audit adjustment for this, but the hospital will have positioned itself to take advantage of a favorable court ruling, should one occur.

Some hospitals have reclassified labor room revenue and expense to outpatient. If a room has not been assigned, there is some justification to stating that labor room services occur before admission. However, care must be taken to ensure there will be no corresponding reduction in collections from commercial insurance companies that do not pay for outpatient services. If this is properly structured, there should be no loss of revenue from private payers.

Chapter 8

Determination of Reimbursement

To maximize reimbursement on the settlement forms, the hospital must consider which limits it may exceed. All of the work performed up to this point is futile if one of the limits is exceeded. However, if the hospital has prepared adequately, it will find it relatively easy to complete the settlement schedules. (Current Medicare forms and instructions relating to the determination of reimbursement are contained in Appendix F. These should be reviewed in conjunction with this chapter to gain a better understanding of the techniques discussed.)

PREPARATION FOR SETTLEMENT

Appealed Items

The hospital should take on its cost report all items that are currently being appealed by the hospital industry. At this writing, the list of appealed issues includes, but is not limited to, the following:

- Labor room days are required to be included in the midnight census.
- Medicare does not allow normal bad debt expense.
- Medicare does not allow charity care expense. The new regulations specifically disallow this, but it will continue to be argued in the courts.
- Medicare requires malpractice insurance to be directly apportioned.
- Medicare does not allow return on equity for tax-exempt institutions.
- Medicare principles depart from GAAP in numerous circumstances.
- Appeal items that are unique to a particular institution.

The hospital is required to disclose the fact that items relating to the above issues were treated differently on the cost report than they are in the regulations. There is also a requirement that the amount of reimbursement in dispute be disclosed.

It is often advantageous to file two cost reports. The first would be a signed cost report with all the appealed items included. The second would not be signed and would be prepared according to the regulations. The unsigned report would not be official but it would facilitate the desk audit and interim settlement.

On all appealed items and other controversial items that the hospital has treated differently from the regulations or instructions, the hospital should have a file of documentation. A letter to the Medicare Bureau under the Freedom of Information Act, requesting all documentation on a particular regulation or instruction, often produces documentation that reveals weaknesses in the government position or indicates items that can be used in an appeal. The Medicare Bureau is required to respond to requests under the Freedom of Information Act. There is a nominal charge for photocopies, but the value of the information normally far exceeds the cost.

Other documentation for this file would include copies of sections from the health insurance manuals, material from the Commerce Clearing House, copies of the exact wording of the applicable regulations, documentation from the intermediary, and internal notes and schedules. A separate file on all items that are likely to be disputed on the cost report makes research easier and more effective.

The Data Base

Limits are now based primarily on a hospital's case mix. Hospitals should request a copy of the file used by the Medicare Bureau to develop its case mix index. This can then be used in developing strategies to maximize reimbursement. If they are not already together, the medical records and the billing file data should be combined. The combined file can then be used to develop profitability by case type, to track case mix changes, and to document exception requests.

Anything that can change the case mix index or that can be called unique to a hospital should be documented. The appeals that are won are those that are the best documented. If the hospital attracts a new physician, that physician's cases should be carefully studied for at least a year to determine the case mix index. The index for the physician can then be compared to the average for the hospital.

HOSPITAL COST LIMITS

The Limit of the Lower of Cost or Charges

The secretary of HHS can repeal or reinstate the limit of the lower of cost or charges at the secretary's discretion. This limit states that, if the hospital's normal charge is less than cost as determined for Medicare, the hospital will receive only its customary charge. Historically, this limit has had little impact on reimbursement. Any amounts disallowed are carried forward to future cost reports, and the institution merely has to raise prices to eliminate the offset.

A new provider can carry disallowed costs forward for five years rather than the customary two years. Therefore, if the hospital undergoes a corporate reorganization, is sold, or is leased, it may be advantageous to obtain a new provider number. Obtaining a new provider number is also advantageous in working with other limits.

Section-223 Limits

Beginning with the fiscal year starting July 1, 1974, Medicare has established limits on hospital costs. From 1974 through 1982, these limits applied only to routine service costs. For cost reporting periods beginning on or after October 1, 1972, the limits were expanded to include all hospital operating costs except malpractice insurance costs, nursing school costs, approved intern/resident costs, and capital-related costs. Prior to 1982, hospitals attempted to transfer costs from routine service to ancillary departments; since 1982, hospitals should attempt to transfer costs to capital, nursing schools, and intern/resident service.

The Section-223 limitation was to be applied on an average-cost, per case basis, adjusted for the institution's case mix complexity. For the first year, the limit is set at 120 percent of the mean for hospitals of the same type; for the second year, the limit was 115 percent of the mean; for the third and subsequent years, the limit was 110 percent of the mean. In April of 1983 the law was changed to eliminate Section-223 limits for cost report years beginning after October of 1983. These limits have been replaced with a system to phase in prospective payments. Although the Section-223 limits have been eliminated, the secretary of HHS was given broad authority to ensure that payments under prospective payment will not exceed the amount that would have been paid under these limits.

It is expected that HHS's annual adjustment for inflation will be conservative. The hospital should calculate its own inflation estimate in order to be prepared to request an exception. This is especially important if patient acuity is increased because of new technology, recruitment of specialists, shorter lengths of stay, or more procedures performed on an outpatient basis.

The severity of a hospital stay is determined according to the ICD-9-CM code. It is important to ensure that medical records place as high a classification as possible on each Medicare and Medicaid discharge. This is especially important if the patient is admitted for multiple purposes. If the hospital exceeds the limit, it can file for an exception based on patient acuity as determined by more complex discharge codes.

Target Rate Reimbursement

In addition to expanded Section-223 limits, the Tax Equity and Fiscal Responsibility Act of 1982 (TEFRA) also introduced a target rate limit. In 1983, hospitals and other providers, therefore, receive the least of:

- cost as defined by Medicare
- customary charges (unless HHS chooses to temporarily repeal this)
- Section-223 limits, which compares a hospital to other similar hospitals for 1983
- target rate reimbursement, which compares a hospital with itself in prior years.

Target rate reimbursement uses the same cost as the case mix rate. It is an all-inclusive rate based on discharges. The base year for a hospital's target is the cost report year beginning on or after October 1, 1981. For most institutions, this is the fiscal year ending in 1982. It is therefore important that this year contain as many costs as possible and that its cost report contain as many reimbursement maximization techniques as possible. There is no provision in the regulations to adjust case-mix costs other than through filing a cost report.

If a particular reimbursement technique was not used, a hospital should attempt to re-open its 1982 cost report or attempt to add costs to it before final settlement. In reopening the 1982 report, attempts should be made to add expenses to the general ledger. This includes expensing warranty costs on new equipment as well as training costs. If the hospital has not adopted LIFO inventory valuation, 1982 is the best year to make this change. No approval is needed to adopt LIFO inventory valuation, and it significantly adds to expenses, especially in the first year. Any renovations that were capitalized should be examined. For 1982 only, it may be advantageous to shift as many outpatient expenses to inpatient, regardless of how this affects 1982 reimbursement. All of the reimbursement techniques discussed in earlier chapters are especially important as applied to 1982.

The target rate of reimbursement is applicable to the first three cost reporting periods after October 1, 1982. For most hospitals, these are the fiscal years ending in 1983, 1984, and 1985. The target rate will be the 1982 operating cost per case increased by the percentage increase in the hospital wage and price index, plus one percentage point. A hospital with costs above the target rate will receive 25 percent of the amount above the target in 1983 and 1984 and no more than the target rate in 1985.

An exception can be granted for changes in the case mix and for other unusual circumstances. Hospitals should carefully monitor changes in their case mix as well as the accuracy of their classification of patient discharge diagnoses.

Other Limits

There is presently a limit on purchased therapy services, including respiratory therapy, physical therapy, and other services. The limit is based on government calculations for wages and wage increases. However, hospitals should not assume that the government calculations are correct. If the hospital loses reimbursement because of a limit, it should perform its own wage rate study and, if it is advantageous, file for an exception. This would be especially appropriate for a group appeal if a region or area with several hospitals has lost reimbursement because of the therapy limits.

For provider-based physicians, there is a new billing screen equal to 60 percent of the screens for physicians in an office setting. This limit assumes that 40 percent of a nonprovider-based physician's costs are overhead. It may be advantageous for a hospital to offer billing services for physicians but not do combined billing. This technique would be even more beneficial if the hospital underwent a corporate reorganization and had a sister corporation perform the billing service. For most hospital-based physicians, the overhead rate will be far less than 40 percent. Additional funds spent to classify physicians as nonhospital-based may be exceeded by the additional reimbursement. This is especially likely in a high-cost reimbursed hospital.

Effective on or after October 1, 1982, reimbursement for inpatient services that are furnished by radiologists and pathologists who accept assignment for those services is reduced from 100 percent to 80 percent. This increases beneficiary coinsurance requirements because coinsurance payers must pay the 20 percent. This provision will very significantly affect billing and cashiering cost. It will also increase Part-B bad debts that are not reimbursed by Medicare. Hospitals thus should consider renegotiating contracts for radiology and pathology services in order to eliminate, or at least minimize, the reimbursement effect.

Beginning with cost reporting periods starting on or after October 1, 1982, Medicare imposes a cost reduction for hospitals that have both private and semiprivate room accommodations. This penalty is to eliminate what the government calls a private room subsidy. The cost penalty is calculated on a ratio of prices for private rooms versus prices for semiprivate rooms. Hospitals thus may find it advantageous to reduce the price spread between private and semiprivate rooms. If the difference is very small, the private room penalty will be very small. However, these savings must be evaluated against the loss in income from collection of the higher rate for private rooms from non-Medicare patients.

STRATEGIES TO REDUCE THE IMPACT OF LIMITS

Capital-Related Costs

Capital-related costs are specifically excluded from most Medicare limits. These costs are culled out, and only costs net of capital are subject to limits.

The hospital should have a long-range capital cost specifically planned to reduce operating costs. New equipment requires less personnel time than old equipment. New buildings are more efficient and require less personnel to maintain, to clean, and to service patients than old buildings. New equipment also requires fewer repairs than old equipment. Money spent on automation is not subject to limits.

As ceilings and limits become more prevalent, inefficient hospitals will not receive full reimbursement. If a hospital is at a limit, it may be beneficial to purchase automation or other capital items just to reduce operating costs. Since existing equipment represents a sunk cost, it is immaterial whether it is still useful or not.

If the hospital has a high percentage of cost payer patients or if the hospital is at a cost limit, its buildings should be phased out as they become inefficient. For some institutions, the only way to survive is to spend millions of dollars on capital-related cost to reduce operating cost.

If the hospital anticipates time delays in the certificate-of-need process, or if there is a possibility that the certificate of need will not be approved, an attempt should be made to split the project into several projects, with each less than the current certificate-of-need limit. Renovations and remodeling performed by the hospital's maintenance staff should be expensed up to the point where the hospital is over one of the cost limits. After that point, an attempt should be made to capitalize work performed by the maintenance staff.

The certificate-of-need process has also been successfully avoided through corporate reorganization. Only health care institutions must receive a certificate of need for capital purchases. Through a corporate reorganization, one of the hospital's sister corporations can purchase the needed equipment without a review process. (Corporate reorganizations are discussed in the next chapter.)

Target Rate

New hospitals and risk-basis HMOs are exempt from target rate limits. Therefore, if possible, it would be advantageous for a hospital to obtain a new provider number. Hospitals that undertake a corporate reorganization, build a replacement facility, or are taken over by a chain should investigate this possibility.

A hospital should not allow the bonus or penalty of target rate reimbursement to affect current operating cost to the point where it cannot sustain that cost over a long period of time. The target rate provisions of TEFRA were originally intended to cover three years. However, the provision for a bonus expires after the first year and cost reimbursement will be phased out over four years. There is no way to tell what will be imposed after the three-year target rate reimbursement limit expires. It is possible that the Medicare Bureau will use the costs achieved in the third year or the lowest cost achieved over the three-year period as a basis for further target reimbursement limits. If the hospital has achieved a low operating cost in order to achieve a bonus but is operating at an expense level that cannot be sustained, this will severely penalize its reimbursement.

To calculate the effect of the savings or the penalty, the hospital can use the following bonus formulas:

$$BP = TC - AC$$

where BP = Bonus potential
TC = Target costs per discharge
AC = Actual costs per discharge

$$B = \frac{BP \times PM}{2}$$

where B = Bonus
BP = Bonus potential
PM = Percentage of patient revenue that is Medicare

To illustrate, assume that a hospital has achieved a level of expenditures per case that is $100,000 below the target costs. The hospital has total reimbursement of $10.0 million and its target costs allow reimbursement of $10.1 million. Assume further that the hospital is 50-percent Medicare reimbursed. Thus:

$$BP = \$10.1 \text{ million} - \$10.0 \text{ million}$$
$$BP = \$100,000$$
$$B = \frac{\$100,000 \times 0.50}{2}$$
$$B = \$25,000$$

In this case, the hospital has reduced expenses by $100,000 and received only $25,000 from Medicare. Unless the hospital was inefficient or wasteful prior to 1982, it would be difficult to achieve $100,000 in permanent cost savings. There is no longer a provision for a bonus after the first year.

Penalty Formula

If a hospital exceeds the target rate of cost per discharge, it is reimbursed for 25 percent of the excess up to the Section-223 limit in the first and second year. In the third year, there is no reimbursement for excess. The first two years for most hospitals are fiscal years ending in 1983 and 1984. The third year for most hospitals is 1985. At this writing, it is difficult to determine what the penalty formula will be after 1985.

The formula for computing a penalty in the first and second year is:

$$PP = AC - TC$$
and
$$P = PP \times MP \times .75$$
where: PP = Potential penalty
   AC = Actual costs per discharge
   TC = Target costs per discharge
   P = Penalty
   MP = Percentage of patient revenue that is Medicare

To illustrate, assume a hospital's actual costs per discharge times the number of discharges equals $10.1 million. Assume further that the target rate allows costs of $10 million and that 50 percent of the patient revenue is Medicare. The penalty is:

$$PP = \$10.1 \text{ million} - \$10.0 \text{ million} = \$100,000$$
$$P = \$100,000 \times .50 \times .75 = \$37,500$$

The hospital has lost $37,500. In the third year the loss would be $50,000. Thus, the hospital has already lost hundreds of thousands of additional dollars on its Medicare and Medicaid patients. This additional loss is added to the existing allowance for contractual allowances that the hospital attempts to pass on to insurance companies in its pricing strategy.

Target rate reimbursement should be monitored. However, administrators and boards should not allow this to intimidate them into cutting needed expenditures from the budget.

Target rate reimbursement excludes capital costs and education costs. Expenditures that can be capitalized will increase reimbursement. Costs that can be transferred to outpatient, intern/resident programs or to schools of nursing will improve reimbursement. If the hospital is already below the target rate of cost, it must weigh the benefit of obtaining a bonus in 1983 against the uncertainty of what the regulations will be after 1985.

Accounting Techniques

The most important accounting techniques are those that gather information that may be used to request an exception. This includes data on local economic conditions that may be used to prove a classification at variance with the Medicare Bureau. It also includes data to support atypical costs for any reason. The Medicare Bureau's most common classification errors are those on per capita income and salary costs.

It may be advantageous to establish new revenue and expense cost centers. This can cull out an activity in an existing cost center that is highly cost reimbursed. Pricing on the activity can then be set on the new center to retain a profit.

The government will not pay for expenses associated with union campaigns. It is important, therefore, to classify outside consultants' fees in such a manner as to preclude them being called union expenses.

It has been proposed that, after 1985, Medicare reimburse hospitals based totally on diagnostic-related groupings (DRGs). The use of reimbursement techniques to minimize the effect of DRG reimbursement has not been explored. However, to prepare for the possibility of a DRG-based method of reimbursement, hospitals should begin to gather cost data based on DRG.

Blue Cross Cost Reports

As hospitals reach the new limits imposed by Medicare, there will be more cost shifting to insurance companies and other payers. In approximately half of the states, Blue Cross reimburses hospitals according to a cost report rather than on a billed charge basis. In many of the states in which Blue Cross reimburses on billed charges, there is a contract with the hospital defining how payment will be made.

It is important to scrutinize all proposals by Blue Cross to change its contract with the hospital. This is true for states in which Blue Cross pays a percentage of billed charges as well as for states in which Blue Cross reimburses according to a cost contract. If the provisions of the proposed new contract are not favorable to the hospital, it should not be signed.

It is also increasingly important to review changes in Blue Cross cost reporting forms. If the new forms contain provisions for changes in Medicare regulations, the hospital should determine whether the contract requires this. Often Blue Cross plans will change their cost reports when major changes are made in Medicare regulations. If, however, there has been no change in the contract, the hospital may effectively ignore the new cost reporting forms. This can be accomplished by using the old, outdated cost report forms or by substituting hospital-prepared schedules for the schedules included in the cost report package.

OBTAINING EXCEPTIONS

Exceptions to reimbursement rules can be granted by the intermediary or the Medicare Bureau. If the intermediary or Medicare Bureau does not approve the request for an exception, the hospital may obtain it from the PRRB or in the district courts. Exception requests submitted through the courts are often more effective as well as less expensive if they are made on behalf of several hospitals in a group appeal.

Case Limits

The regulations provide for exceptions to the case limits for the following reasons:

- atypical services
- extraordinary circumstances
- fluctuating population
- medical/paramedical education
- unusual labor costs
- essential community hospital services
- changes in case mix
- hospitals with a disproportionate share of Medicare or Medicaid patients
- psychiatric hospitals

An atypical service can be whatever the hospital defines as such in an exception request. Almost every hospital has something that is unique. Hospitals should develop the relevant costs and statistics at an early time to support possible exception requests. Internally generated cost studies, long-form audit statements, board minutes, and other similar information should not be shared with the intermediary. In requesting an exception for atypical services, it is best if the intermediary does not have information that could be used to dispute the hospital's claims.

Exception requests based on fluctuating population require demographic information that is readily available from the Census Bureau. Projections of future population demographics are made by universities, state economic units, and other organizations. To prepare for an exception, the hospital should perform admission studies at least twice a year to define the primary and secondary service area.

Exception requests arising from unusual labor costs require that the hospital have data on increases in average hourly pay rates due to acuity and technology advances. The additions to hospital payroll are normally skilled, highly educated personnel. When the hospital acquires a new technology, the wages of the personnel needed to perform the new service should be documented. Average hourly pay rates have increased, and will continue to increase, due to patient acuity and new services. Trends toward doing more procedures on an outpatient basis and toward shorter lengths of stay are having profound effects on nursing, technicians, and other highly paid personnel, but very little effect on housekeeping or laundry personnel.

It is anticipated that changes in case mix will represent the largest number of exception requests. However, it is recommended that all requests contain several reasons. Changes in case mix can be combined with unusual labor costs, a fluctuating population, and other reasons in a single exception request.

The case mix index is based on a 20-percent sample for calendar year 1980. A hospital can submit a request to correct its limits up to 180 days after the end of the first year in which the limits apply. The government will then adjust the index upward or downward. Each hospital should obtain a copy of its data that are used by Medicare to establish its case mix index. After studying these data, if it appears a higher index is attainable, a request for a review should be made.

Target Rate Limits

The target rate limits have two possible exemptions and two possible exceptions. The hospital is exempt if it is a new hospital or a risk-basis HMO. Procurement of a new provider number because of a corporate reorganization, a takeover by a chain, or for some other reason will exempt a hospital from the target rate limits. However, requests for a new provider number should not be made if significant expense reductions are being planned, because the new provider number would preclude earning a bonus for achieving a cost per discharge that is less than the target rate.

As noted, the regulations provide for exceptions because of extraordinary circumstances or changes in case mix. In filing for an exception to the case mix limits, a concurrent request for an adjustment to the target rate should be made. The hospital should monitor significant and abrupt changes in organization, range of service, medical specialty, or other relevant, identifiable event. To file for a target rate exception, the hospital must submit 100 percent of its discharge data for the current period. This must be submitted within 180 days of the settlement date.

Chapter 9

Corporate Reorganization

The health care environment has changed dramatically over the years. Most of this change has been brought about by the government. One of the major areas of change has been in organizational structure. In this chapter, we examine the conditions that have led to hospital corporate reorganizations, look at some of the resulting benefits, and describe likely future trends.

BACKGROUND

Before Medicare

Until 1945, the federal and state governments remained totally out of health care. Communities, religious groups, and other private groups constructed and maintained hospitals. Hospital boards held regular fund-raising events to construct new buildings and to provide care for the poor and elderly. Hospital care was inexpensive, but by today's standards it was also unsophisticated.

By 1945, the mood of the federal government was changing. It was felt that the government had a responsibility to solve the problems of its people in a more direct manner. Hospitals were becoming more sophisticated, and construction costs were soaring. Communities could no longer raise enough capital to build or improve their hospitals.

In 1945, the Hill-Burton Act was passed to pay for construction and renovation of American hospitals. The program allocated more than $10 billion in over 7,000 projects. Almost every American hospital and virtually every community received Hill-Burton funds. The federalization of health care had begun.

By 1960, it was clear that new or improved facilities were not enough to solve the health care needs of the poor and the elderly. Many citizens could not afford the cost of care. Pressure began to build for the government to become more involved in health care delivery.

Existing medical schools were upgraded and new medical schools were built with federal incentives. Between 1960 and 1980, the number of medical school graduates more than doubled. In 1965, the Medicare Act was passed, and in 1967 the government began to pay directly for health care. Also, about the same time, expensive advances in health care technology began to grow at an alarming rate.

The Medicare Program

When Medicare was first introduced, many physicians, administrators, and hospital boards believed that it did not represent an appropriate role for the government. To overcome this resistance, the government made it very attractive for hospitals and physicians to participate. For hospital care, the program paid costs, plus a 2-percent allowance over costs. Physicians were paid charges on a class of patients who represented collection risks because they were unemployed and often poor. Medicaid was started to provide health care for the poor. It was financially attractive for hospitals to participate in the Medicaid program, because the patients under the program had a very high charge-off rate.

Beginning about 1974, it became clear that the Medicare and Medicaid program was creating serious financial burdens on state and local governments and was straining the national economy. The government had gone from no involvement in health care, to almost 30 years of increasing involvement as a friend of health care, to a point where it now had to attempt to restrict health care growth. Throughout this period, the country was producing an increasing number of physicians, and medical technology was advancing rapidly.

An Adversary Relationship

In 1974, the Public Health Planning Act was passed. Health planning was to be done on a state-by-state basis with federal guidelines. Significant capital expenditures by a "health facility" required certificate-of-need approval. Hospital boards could no longer make capital decisions on their own.

Beginning in the mid-1970s, the Medicare and Medicaid programs became more restrictive. In order to control government expenditures, hospitals and others were paid less than cost. The process was slow at first, and hospitals compensated by charging private-pay patients more. The private insurance companies passed the cost on through higher premiums.

As the Medicare and Medicaid programs paid less than cost to hospitals, disputes over the interpretation of the regulations defining allowable costs became commonplace. Hospitals across the country went to court with the Medicare Bureau over cost reports. Today, the government is clearly in an adversary relationship with the health care industry.

Competition and the IRS

As for-profit hospital chains became larger and more powerful, their presence created competition for tax-exempt hospitals and put pressure on the IRS to examine the actions of tax-exempt hospitals. Before the existence of the for-profit hospital chains, there was no reason for the IRS to involve itself in health care. The IRS regulations developed over a long period of time and were influenced by large industrial corporations. The Medicare regulations developed over a short period of time and were influenced by the government's need to restrain its budget.

The IRS regulations follow GAAP relatively closely; Medicare regulations make wide departures from GAAP. Because the IRS is a part of the Treasury Department and the Medicare Bureau is a part of HHS, the differences in policies and attitudes of the two agencies are numerous.

The competition brought about by the presence of the for-profit hospital chains also brought regulation of hospitals by antitrust agencies and other regulatory departments of the government. Many of the regulations promulgated by the IRS and other government agencies are counterproductive to the goals of the Medicare Bureau and in direct conflict with Medicare regulations.

EXPERIENCE OF OTHER INDUSTRIES

Other industries have responded to government pressures through corporate restructuring. This section examines the parallels with the current trend toward hospital corporate restructuring.

The Banking Industry

Throughout the 1970s, banking in America became increasingly more competitive. As individual banks attempted to become more aggressive in marketing, banking regulations created a barrier. To avoid the banking regulations, bank boards formed bank-holding companies. This allowed the banks to market nontraditional services and to create bank chains controlled or owned by a central holding company.

As hospital regulations become more restrictive, hospitals are also creating new corporate structures that allow them to market nontraditional services. This corporate restructuring is also creating hospital chains that are owned or controlled by health care holding companies. These companies are involved in health care in hospitals, wellness clinics, health services in factories, educational programs, hospices, professional office buildings, and other areas. They are not just hospitals; they have larger missions and purposes.

Colleges and Universities

Colleges and universities found that, as they successfully solicited funds from alumni and others, there was a corresponding reduction in their appropriations from state legislatures and other sponsors. But alumni had little incentive to give to their alma mater if there was no net increase in the amount of money available to the university. To solve this problem, most alumni created independent foundations to accept donations and gifts. These foundations used their funds to purchase equipment, to fund professorships, to construct buildings and to assist the university in other ways.

As hospitals successfully created new sources of revenue or accepted donations, they also found reductions in their allowable rate increases from state rate-setting agencies or in their cost reimbursement. There was no incentive for hospitals to seek new revenue sources or to solicit donations because the net amount of funds available to the organization was not thereby increased.

To solve this problem, many hospitals formed foundations. In the beginning, these foundations were very successful in fulfilling their purpose. Then Medicare regulations began to negate the benefits gained from controlled foundations. As a result, some hospitals created noncontrolled foundations. Other boards were not willing to create independent foundations because they did not want to lose control.

Before the mid-1970s, hospital foundations were able to solve adequately the problems of hospitals. At this writing, however, they provide only a partial solution to most of the problems created by health care regulations.

Other Industries

Since the 1900s, American corporations have been undergoing corporate restructuring to take advantage of tax laws, to avoid restrictive regulations, to become more competitive, and to pursue other goals. In this connection, it should be remembered that a corporation's legal structure often has nothing in common with its management structure. There are highly decentralized legal structures with centralized management and control systems; there are also highly centralized legal structures with decentralized management and control systems. As the environment changes, corporations continue to change their legal structures in an unending, evolving process.

In this trend, hospital corporations are responding appropriately to regulations by undergoing corporate restructuring. As in other areas, there are centralized hospital legal structures with decentralized management and control systems, and there are also decentralized hospital legal structures with centralized management and control systems. As regulations, competitive pressures, and other factors change, health care corporations continue to change their legal structures.

Though, as we have noted, there is no necessary correlation between changes in an organization's legal structure and changes in its management structure (since the reasons for change in the two areas are often different), most changes in an organization's legal structure bring about corresponding changes in its management structure. The decisions affecting the two aspects are the responsibility of the board of directors.

As indicated, hospitals throughout the United States are examining the benefits of corporate reorganization as an appropriate and timely response to the problems of overregulation. As in other industries, since the mid-1970s it has become increasingly advantageous for hospitals to form new legal structures. Many knowledgeable observers believe that, by the year 2000, all American hospitals will either have become part of a large chain or will be operating under new and evolving legal structures.

THE PRESENT ENVIRONMENT

Reimbursement Maximization

In this section, our discussion of the principles of reimbursement maximization relates to Medicare regulations. However, most of these principles are also applicable to Medicaid reimbursement and, in those states where hospitals are cost reimbursed by Blue Cross, to Blue Cross reimbursement.

As Medicare regulations erode a hospital's financial base, the board often seeks new sources of revenue or ways to cut cost. In many cases, income from new sources of income is offset on the hospital's cost reports against expenses. In other instances, expensive hospital overhead is allocated to a new revenue cost center, and then the cost center is disallowed on the cost report. In both cases, the hospital's reimbursement is reduced, and new sources of revenue do not benefit the institution.

Before a hospital develops new sources of revenue, it should investigate corporate restructuring. To maximize reimbursement, an attempt should be made to put all nonreimbursable cost centers and low reimbursable cost centers into a corporation that is distinct from the hospital corporation. This is easier to accomplish if the cost center being spun off is physically separate from the hospital.

The hospital should also attempt to place all new, nonacute, inpatient care health services in a corporation that is separate and distinct from the hospital corporation. Because of IRS rulings, this is especially important if the new health service is profitable. With careful planning, the additional cost reimbursement often pays for the cost of the corporate reorganization in a single year.

The Internal Revenue Service

Tax-exempt organizations receive tax-exemptions to perform specific activities. These are outlined in tax-exemption letters issued by district offices of the IRS. Activities not within the scope of an exemption letter are called unrelated business activities and are taxable. Most hospital exemption certificates have a narrow scope, partly because they were issued years ago before anyone envisioned that hospitals would engage in anything other than inpatient hospital care.

In a reorganization, the organization should attempt to create one or more new corporate entities with exemption letters that are as broad as possible. This allows the organization to engage in aggressive new activities under a screen of tax exemption.

In a corporate restructuring, the hospital should create at least one taxable corporate entity. All taxable activities can then be combined into the one for-profit entity. Activities or services that operate at a loss should also be put into the taxable corporation to offset taxable losses against taxable income.

Tax-exempt hospitals must also plan to avoid inurement issues. Inurement occurs when a tax-exempt corporation uses its exempt status to benefit a taxable corporation or an individual. Often, the IRS has ruled inurement even when all parties have benefited in an arms-length transaction. Any activity that could raise the question of inurement should be placed in the taxable corporation or in a tax-exempt corporation other than the hospital. A nonhospital, tax-exempt corporation is normally not as significant as the hospital from either an operating point of view or a public relations point of view. IRS actions against such a tax-exempt corporation will not, therefore, be as damaging.

A final point to consider is the accounting allocation of overhead. On cost reports if there is only one corporation, as little overhead as possible should be allocated to the taxable activity, since it is a nonallowable cost center for Medicare and other cost reimbursement purposes. Notwithstanding cost reports, as much overhead as possible should be allocated to the taxable activity in order to reduce taxable net income. However, the IRS may examine the cost reports, and the Medicare auditors may examine the IRS reports, which can lead to audit adjustments and controversy.

With separate and distinct corporations, overhead allocations can be assigned by written agreements that are designed to gain maximum reimbursement. If they are reasonable, intracompany allocations are normally unchallenged. Intercompany allocations are often ignored by both Medicare and IRS auditors.

Certificate of Need

All major capital expenditures by health care institutions are subject to certificate-of-need (CON) regulations. This does not pertain just to patient-related activities. Professional office buildings, meals on wheels, hospices, schools of nursing, wellness programs, feeder organizations, outpatient clinics, industrial health programs, and other activities that are contemplated by a hospital but may have little or nothing to do with acute inpatient care must be approved by the state health planning agency. Nonhospital-based corporations are not subject to CON legislation. Many organizations successfully avoid CON applications through corporate reorganization. The expenditure in question is simply made by a newly created corporation that is not subject to CON laws.

There are many reasons to avoid the CON process. CON applications are public information; when a CON application is filed, the hospital's plans are made known to competitors and others in minute detail. In acquiring real estate, hundreds of thousands of dollars can often be saved if the facility's plans are not made public. In the competition for new services, the element of surprise can create crucial leverage. Yet hospitals, unlike any other industry in America, must make their plans known to the public and to their competition in minute detail at an early stage.

Another reason to attempt to avoid the CON process is the cost in time and money. The CON process is a complicated and expensive process and often takes over a year. In the time required to obtain CON approval, inflation can add thousands of dollars to the cost of a project. The CON process also requires management time that cannot be used to solve other problems.

It should also be noted that not all CON applications are approved. If subjected to the process, there is a risk that the hospital may not be allowed to proceed with its plans. Corporations that are not subject to CON legislation are not subject to this risk. Thus, an attempt to avoid the CON process through corporate restructuring is an appropriate, prudent, and timely response to government regulation.

Rate Setting

Over half of the states have some form of rate-setting legislation. Many of the states that do not have rate setting at this time will have it in the near future. In addition, there is always the possibility of national rate-setting legislation in the future.

If a hospital builds feeder clinics or offers other services that produce a net profit, the rate-setting agency can consider this profit when approving rates. The effect might be to negate the hospital's effort to accumulate capital for needed capital improvements or for other reasons. In this case, there would be no reason to do anything about the erosion of the financial base caused by the loss from Medicare and Medicaid patients.

If there is a loss on a new service, the rate-setting agency can elect to ignore the loss when approving hospital rates. It can ignore nonacute care losses on several grounds. The hospital is then faced with an operating loss and no way to recover that loss. However, if the new service or activity had been properly placed in a separate corporation, there would have been no offset.

Capital Accumulation

The hospitals that survive will be those who have accumulated capital. Without capital, a hospital cannot replace old facilities, keep up with technology fast enough to ensure the loyalty of its medical staff, or offer competitive new services. Yet the present regulatory environment prohibits hospitals from accumulating capital and erodes the existing financial base. If the hospital attempts to acquire capital through cost reductions, its cost reimbursement is reduced. If it attempts to raise capital through price increases, it finds that cost payers ignore price increases and that there is a heavy Hill-Burton charity requirement. If it attempts to accumulate revenues by developing new services, the profits of the new ventures are confiscated through cost reimbursement or rate setting. In addition, new sources of revenue bring new IRS headaches.

If a hospital does accumulate capital, interest earned on the funds is normally offset on the cost report. Yet accumulated interest earnings are a way of protecting a capital base in inflationary times. For example, if one kept a million dollars for ten years and inflation was eight percent per year, the purchasing power of the fund would have shrunk to $463,400. However, if the funds had been invested at the eight-percent inflation rate, they would be worth the same at the end of ten years as in the base year. Normally, funds are invested at approximately two percent above the current inflation rate. Thus, if a hospital could protect funds from interest offset, it would gain rather than lose purchasing power.

The most effective way for a hospital to accumulate funds is through a corporate restructuring in which a corporate entity other than the hospital earns, accumulates, and invests the funds. By putting activities outside of the regulatory environment in which American hospitals must operate, otherwise unrealized corporate goals can often be accomplished.

Access to Capital Markets

The capital markets are controlled by investment bankers, who are assumed to be sophisticated, perceptive, intelligent, and competitive. They understand the regulatory environment in which hospitals operate. Because of applicable regulations, a provider in the hospital industry receives lower ratings on its bond issues than a company with a financial statement of similar strength in another industry. The lower rating means that the hospital must pay a higher interest rate. Thus, because of the current competition in the hospital environment, many hospitals have been denied access to the capital markets; they cannot borrow funds at any interest rate.

The capital market favors organizations that have responded to a changing environment with new sources of revenue, new services, hospital chains, or shared services. This is both predictable and appropriate. With a corporate restructuring and the assistance of an investment banker, the hospital can gain better access to the bond markets at more favorable rates. Technology will continue to drive construction costs higher. Competitive forces will continue to grow and, given the strength of the for-profit chains, will continue to change. At the same time, the regulations will continue to become more prevalent. For many hospitals, access to the capital markets will mean the difference between bankruptcy, getting by with the least amount of discredit, or becoming strong, financially viable institutions.

KINDS OF CORPORATE STRUCTURES

Single Corporations

The traditional single corporate entity has been the dominant corporate structure adopted by American hospitals over the years. Since hospitals were nearly always tax-exempt, until the advent of Medicare, there was no reason to consider anything more complex. However, regulations and competition have made the single corporate entity no longer appropriate for many hospitals. With this model, it is difficult to maximize reimbursement or create new revenue sources. Many hospital experts believe that, by the year 2000, the single hospital corporate entity will be nonexistent, or at least very rare. They believe that hospitals will either become parts of hospital chains or will be corporations within a local health care holding company involved in many nontraditional activities.

Controlled Corporations

A hospital corporation can create one or more corporate subsidiaries that are controlled by the hospital, as shown in Figure 9–1. This form of corporate structure is a partial solution to environmental pressures. However, GAAP require that all subsidiary financial statements be consolidated with that of the parent corporation. Thus, Medicare, Medicaid, some Blue Cross plans, and some rate-setting agencies will consider only the consolidated financial statements. In such cases, all of the problems associated with reimbursement for the single corporation persist.

This structure does encourage new sources of revenue, eliminates most IRS problems, and gains better access to the capital markets. In it, capital accumulation problems are partially, but not totally, eliminated.

Noncontrolled Corporations

A hospital may create a new not-for-profit corporation that does not have overlapping board members and is not directly controlled by the hospital. Once 501(C)(3) tax-exempt status has been obtained for the new corporation, the present hospital can transfer funds, real estate, and other assets to it. This corporate structure is depicted in Figure 9–2. In this case, the hospital has indirect control over the new health corporation when it is established because it can choose the first board of directors. Thereafter, it can exert influence by having one voting member or an ex officio member on the board of the new corporation. Over a period of years, however, as

Figure 9–1 Controlled Corporations

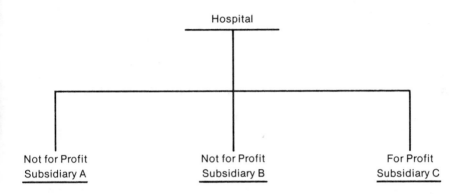

board members are replaced, the hospital may lose control of its health corporation.

The noncontrolled corporate structure solves all of the regulatory and competitive environment problems. Reimbursement can be effectively maximized, IRS problems are eliminated, capital can be accumulated, and the organization can gain better access to the capital markets. In addition, this corporate structure can be changed or adjusted to provide maximum flexibility in response to future regulations and pressures.

The main disadvantage of this model is in the loss of control. The present hospital board may be concerned that the board of the new corporation will not have the wisdom and prudence that the present hospital board has. They may be concerned that the new corporation will compete with the present hospital in marketing new services.

Yet, from a legal and accounting point of view, the noncontrolled corporate structure is the simplest and most effective of the various models.

Figure 9–2 Noncontrolled Corporations

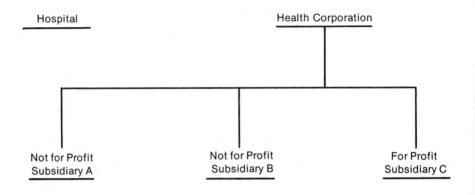

Though the prospect of loss of control has made it unacceptable to many boards, other boards have survived successfully with the noncontrolled corporate structure.

Holding Companies

To establish a holding company structure, a 501(C)(3) tax-exempt corporation is created. The board of the present hospital moves up to become the board of the holding company, and the hospital becomes a subsidiary of the holding company. This structure is shown in Figure 9–3. The board of the hospital can be the same as the board of the holding company, or a separate board for the hospital can be appointed. At least one of the newly formed corporations is for-profit, as in the other models.

Figure 9–3 Holding Company

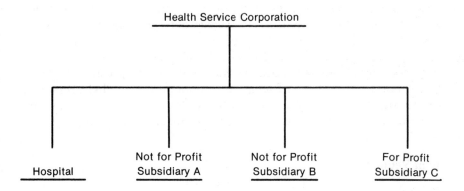

The holding company structure avoids all of the indicated IRS problems, allows the organization to enter into new competitive markets, permits accumulation of capital, and solves the rate-review issue. However, it only partially solves the cost reimbursement problems because the holding company is considered a related organization according to Medicare and Medicaid regulations. There are some problems associated with determining the cost of services provided by the related organization; and, in most instances, the holding company is not allowed to make a reasonable profit on services provided to the hospital.

Some of the advantages of the holding company structure are that:

• It is easier to add new acute care hospitals and to form a hospital chain.

- The structure affords slightly better access to the capital markets compared to the noncontrolled corporation model.
- It is easier to retain control.

The holding company model is currently the most popular form of structure chosen by hospitals that are undergoing corporate reorganization. It allows for a great deal of flexibility in adjusting to changing regulations and changing competitive environments.

This model is similar to the controlled corporation model. The major difference is that the hospital is a subsidiary of a corporation and does not have any subsidiary corporations of its own. Financial statements are consolidated upward but not downward. The financial statements of the parent corporation do not appear on the statements of a subsidiary. Therefore, all of the advantages of separate corporations apply. In its reporting to the Medicare Bureau and the IRS, the hospital need not show the activities of any of the other corporations of the holding company.

Joint Ventures

In a joint venture, two or more hospitals jointly create a new corporation. The newly formed corporation obtains a 501(C)(3) tax exemption. The original hospitals transfer agreed-upon funds, real estate, and other assets to the new corporation. The joint venture form of legal structure is shown in Figure 9–4. This corporate structure may be especially appropriate for government hospitals if the political problems can be managed.

Other Legal Structures

Obviously, a single corporate model will not fit all situations. Each hospital has its own unique factors and environment. However, in the corporate restructuring process, one model that is custom designed for the particular situation is likely to emerge. In addition to those we have examined, other models might be considered.

The asset holding company is a structure in which assets are owned by one entity or entities and are leased to a management company. The nonparent center model has no direct lines of authority or control between it and the hospital that created it. In all other respects, it is similar to the joint venture model. The limited partnership model is one in which the hospital contributes to, and becomes a partner in, a specified venture.

Figure 9–4 A Joint Venture

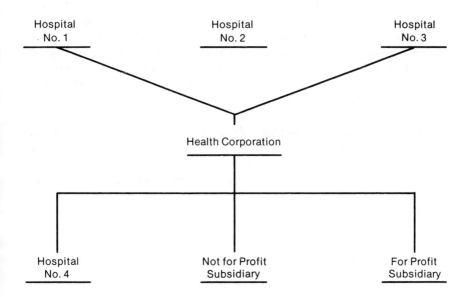

THE REORGANIZATION PROCESS

Reorganization is probably the most effective way to maximize reimbursement today. It is a process that is receiving growing acceptance throughout America.

When To Reorganize

Corporate reorganization is a difficult and complex process. Although the benefits to be gained can be substantial, it should not be done by every hospital. There are two situations in which corporate restructuring can be advantageous. If only one of these situations is present, a study should be made; if both are present, corporate restructuring is a necessity.

The first situation is one in which a hospital performs, or plans to perform, a significant number of activities that cannot be classified as inpatient acute care. These could include maintaining a nursing home, hospice, or professional office building; substantial fund raising; maintaining significant outpatient services; or conducting other nontraditional activities. If the hospital does not perform services other than inpatient acute care, the gains from corporate restructuring may be small.

The second situation is one in which a hospital has an unusually high or a rapidly growing percentage of cost payer patients. Because cost reports allow less than cost, a high number or growing percentage of cost payer patients can destroy the financial base and eventually bankrupt the hospital.

Hospitals that have a relatively low and stable percentage of cost payer patients and do not wish to diversify into new markets would currently gain very little from a corporate restructuring. However, this situation may change in the light of future developments. Under prospective payment the only way to receive payment for new technology may be through a sister corporation.

Restructuring Myths

There are three widespread myths associated with corporate restructuring:

1. The process involves a great deal of risk.
2. It is a new technique, and the hospital should wait to study it.
3. It is not appropriate for government hospitals.

Yet the only risk associated with corporate restructuring is the time, effort, and expense associated with the process. If it is not accepted by Medicare, the IRS, and other relevant entities, the hospital is still no worse off than it was. There is no downside risk, just an upside risk. The chances of a carefully planned restructuring being ignored by others is not very great. Moreover, the process of studying, evaluating, and planning the hospital role and its organizational future is, in itself, an extremely valuable exercise.

The use of corporate restructuring to deal with regulations is not a new technique. The process has been used quite successfully by businesses, banks, and other industrial organizations since the inception of income taxes. And, as we have noted, it has been widely used by American hospitals since the mid-1970s.

Some people believe that communities will not allow free-standing hospitals to disappear. This same thing was said about the neighborhood grocery store and the neighborhood gasoline station. As the environment changes, people change in order to adjust. The stores and service stations that did not adjust to competitive forces at the appropriate time went bankrupt or slowly lost their financial base. In the hospital industry, the presence of the for-profit hospital chains will create more competitive forces. There are thus good reasons to conclude that free-standing community hospitals may disappear if they do not adjust. It is already happening in many communities.

From a legal perspective, it is, in many ways, much easier for a government hospital to undertake a corporate reorganization than it is for a community, not-for-profit hospital to do so. And the ensuing benefits to the government hospital are at least as great, if not greater, than they are to a community hospital. It is only the political problems that are difficult to solve for a city-, county-, or state-owned hospital.

Finally, it should be remembered that exploring the possibility of a corporate reorganization does not necessarily have to lead to that end. A study to investigate the possibility does not necessarily mean that the hospital must undertake the process.

Medicare Regulations Regarding Hospital Cost Reports

The following Medicare instructions apply, at this writing, to preparation of the hospital's Medicare cost report, as discussed in Chapter 2. This appendix is a general overview of the current Medicare cost report.

300. GENERAL

Form HCFA-2552 must be used by all hospitals and hospital-skilled
nursing facility complexes and skilled nursing facilities which
are not hospital based for cost reporting periods beginning on or
after July 1, 1979.

Note that skilled nursing facilities which are not hospital
based must use the identified skilled nursing facility lines and
columns and all appropriate worksheets in determining Medicare
reimbursement in this cost report.

The hospital or hospital-skilled nursing facility complex, or
skilled nursing facility which is not hospital based, may submit
its own forms in lieu of the forms provided. These forms are
acceptable if the forms are approved by the intermediary or HCFA
before being placed into use. (See Chapter 1, section 108, for
the use of substitute cost reporting forms.)

Where substitute cost reporting forms have been accepted for
use, they must be revised and resubmitted for acceptance whenever changes in the law, regulations or program instructions
which have an impact on Medicare cost reporting are adopted.

In addition to Medicare reimbursement, these forms also provide
for the computation of reimbursable hospital and subprovider
component inpatient costs applicable to titles V and XIX. The
worksheets and portions of worksheets applicable to titles V
and XIX should be completed only when reimbursement is being
claimed from these respective programs.

These forms include the step-down method of cost finding
which provides for the allocation of the cost of services
rendered by each general service cost center to other cost
centers which utilize such services. Once the costs of a
general service cost center have been allocated, that cost
center is considered "closed." Being "closed," it will not
receive any of the costs that are substantially allocated from
the remaining general service cost centers. After all costs
of the general service cost centers have been allocated to
the remaining cost centers, the total costs of these remaining
cost centers are further distributed to the departmental
classification to which they pertain, e.g., hospital inpatient,
subprovider inpatient, outpatient.

The double apportionment method of cost finding or a more
sophisticated method of cost finding which is designed to
allocate costs more accurately may be used upon written
approval by the intermediary of a timely request filed in
accordance with the procedures set forth in the PRM, Part I,
chapter 23.

NOTE: Total direct PSRO review costs are not included on
        Worksheet E, Part III, but are shown separately by the
        hospital on form HCFA-152 which must be attached to the
        Medicare cost report.

In completing the worksheets, reductions in expenses must always
be shown in parenthesis (   ).

301.   ROUNDING STANDARDS FOR FRACTIONAL COMPUTATIONS
Throughout the Medicare cost report required computations result
in the use of fractions.   The following is a listing of the worksheets (columns and lines) which require fractional computations
and of the rounding standards to be employed for such computation.

If a residual exists as a result of computing costs using a
fraction, the residual should be included in the largest amount
resulting from the computation.   For example, in cost finding a
unit cost multiplier is applied to the statistics in determining
costs.   After rounding each computation the sum of the allocation
may be more or less than the total cost being allocated.   This
residual should be included in the largest amount resulting from the
allocation.

Worksheet	Page No.	Col(s)	Line(s)	Computation
	3 (Part II)	1-5	7	Percentage - Round to 2 decimal places
	3 (Part III)		2,3 and 7a-7d	Averages - Round to 2 decimal places
	4 (Part IV)	1-4	7	Percentage - Round to 2 decimal places
	4 (Part V)		2,3 and 8a-8d	Averages - Round to 2 decimal places
A-2	7	4	2-5	Ratio - Round to 8 decimal places
A-8-1	13	3 and 5	1-5	Percentage - Round to 2 decimal places
B-1	16 and 17	2-20	74	Ratio - Round to 8 decimal places
C	18	2	2-33	Ratio - Round to 8 decimal places
D-1	21 and 22	4-20	28	Ratio - Round to 8 decimal places

Worksheet	Page No.	Col(s)	Line(s)	Computation
D-1	23	1-4	32 and 40-43	Per Diem - Round to 2 decimal places
D-1	24	1-3	53,56 and 63-67	Per Diem - Round to 2 decimal places
D-2	25 (Part I)	1	3-20	Percentage - Round to 2 decimal places
D-2	25 (Part I)	4	3-12	Per Diem - Round to 2 decimal places
D-2	25 (Part I)	e	17-19	Ratio - Round to 8 decimal places
D-2	25 (Part II)	3	2-10	Per Diem - Round to 2 decimal places
D-3	26	3	1-11	Ratio - Round to 8 decimal places
D-8	27		8-10, 12 and 17-19	Ratio - Round to 8 decimal places
E (Part II)	29		19	Ratio - Round to 8 decimal places
E-2	32	1-4	2 and 15	Ratio - Round to 8 decimal places
E-5 (Part II)	33	1-3	14	Ratio - Round to 8 decimal places
Supp. D-4			3	Ratio - Round to 8 decimal places
Supp. D-5			3	Ratio - Round to 8 decimal places
Supp. F (Part III)	3		3	Ratio - Round to 8 decimal places
Supp. A-8-3	1	2	5-10	Rates - Round to 3 decimal places
Supp. A-8-3	2	1-3	12 and 24	Rate - Round to 3 decimal places

301(Cont.)   FORM HCFA-2552   8-80

Worksheet	Page No.	Col(s)	Line(s)	Computation
Supp. A-8-3	2	1-3	15 and 27	Percentage - Round to 2 decimal places

302. RECOMMENDED SEQUENCE FOR COMPLETING FORM HCFA-2552

Step No.	Worksheet	Page(s)	

PART I - Cost Determination (to be followed by all providers)

Step No.	Worksheet	Page(s)	Computation
1		2	Complete Part I - General except for Certification Statement
2		3	Complete entire page
3		4	Complete entire page
4	A	5	Complete columns 1 through 3, lines 2 through 80
5	A-1 through A-6	6-9	Complete, if applicable
6	A	5	Complete columns 4 and 5, lines 2 through 80
7	A-7	10	Complete lines 1 and 2. If the answer to line 2 is "Yes," lines 3 and 4 should also be completed.
8	A-8	11, 12	Complete lines 1 through 19
9	A-8-1	13	Complete Part A. If the answer to Part A is "Yes," complete Parts B and C
10	Supp. A-8-3	2-3	Complete, if applicable
11	A-8	11, 12	Complete lines 20 through 64
12	A	5	Complete columns 6 and 7, lines 2 through 80
13	A-8-2	13	Complete entire worksheet
14	B and B-1	14-17	Complete entire worksheet

Step No.	Worksheet	Page(s)	

PART II - Departmental Cost Distribution and Cost Apportionment

For Providers Not Using Accommodations Other Than in the Renal Dialysis Department To Furnish Renal Dialysis Services:

1	C	18	Complete entire worksheet
2	D	19	Complete entire worksheet A separate copy of this worksheet must be completed for the hospital, each subprovider, hospital-based skilled nursing facility component or skilled nursing facility.
3	D-1	20-24	Complete Part I (title XVIII /Medicare/) and Part II (titles V and XIX), if applicable
4	D-2	25	Complete only those parts that are applicable. Do not complete Part III unless Parts I and II are completed.
5	D-3	26	Complete entire worksheet
6	Supp. D-4		Complete, if applicable
7	Supp. D-5		Complete, if applicable
8	Supp. D-6		Complete, if applicable

PART III - Departmental Cost Distribution and Cost Apportionment

For Providers Using Accommodations Other Than in the Renal Dialysis Department To Furnish Renal Dialysis Services:

1	C	18	Complete lines 2 through 20, lines 22 and 23, and lines 25 through 33
2	D-1	20-23	Complete Part I
3	Supp. D-7		Complete Part I and/or Part II and Part III, as appropriate

302(Cont.)   FORM HCFA-2552   8-80

Step No.	Worksheet	Page(s)	
4	C	18	Complete lines 21 and 34
5	D	19	Complete entire worksheet. A separate copy of this worksheet must be completed for the hospital, each subprovider, hospital-based skilled nursing facility component or skilled nursing facility.
6	D-1	24	Complete Part II (titles V and XIX), if applicable
7	D-2	25	Complete only those parts that are applicable. Do not complete Part III unless both Parts I and II are completed.
8	D-3	26	Complete entire worksheet
9	Supp. D-4		Complete, if applicable
10	Supp. D-5		Complete, if applicable
11	Supp. D-6		Complete, if applicable

PART IV - Calculation of Reimbursement Settlement

Proprietary Providers:

1	E	29	Complete Part II, lines 7 through 20
2	E-5	33	Complete Part II (titles V and XIX) if applicable, lines 6 through 15
3	D-8	27	Complete entire worksheet
4	E	28	Complete Part I
5	E-5	33	Complete Part I (titles V and XIX), if applicable
6	E-1	31	Complete lines 1 through 4

138 PRINCIPLES OF REIMBURSEMENT IN HEALTH CARE

Step No.	Worksheet	Page(s)	
7	Supp. F	1-3	Complete Part I, lines 1 through 56, Part II and Part III
8	Supp. E-3		Complete, if applicable
9	E	29	Complete Part II, lines 2 through 5; complete lines 21 through 24, as appropriate
10	Title XVIII Supp. E-4		
	or		Complete the appropriate part or parts, if applicable
	Supp. E-4-1		
11	E	30	Complete Part III, lines 1 through 6
12	E-2	32	Complete entire worksheet
13	E	30	Complete Part III, lines 7 through 19
14	E-5	33	Complete Part II, lines 2 through 4; complete line 16 or line 17, as appropriate
15	Titles V & XIX Supp. E-4		
	or		Complete the appropriate part or parts, if applicable
	Supp. E-5		
16	E-5	34	Complete Part III
17	Supp. F	1	Complete Part I, lines 57 through 60
18	G	35	Complete only if maintaining fund type accounting records
19	G-1	36	Provider maintaining fund type accounting records should complete entire worksheet

Step No.	Worksheet	Page(s)	
			Providers not maintaining fund type accounting records should complete only the "General Fund" column
20	G-2	37	Complete entire worksheet
21	G-3	38	Complete entire worksheet
22	Worksheet Checklist	1	Complete entire worksheet
23		2	Complete Certification Statement

PART V - Calculation of Reimbursement Settlement

Nonproprietary Providers and Public Providers Not Rendering Services Free of Charge or at a Nominal Charge:

1	E	29	Complete Part II, lines 7 through 20
2	E-5	33	Complete Part II (titles V and XIX), lines 6 through 15
3	D-8	27	Complete entire worksheet
4	E	28	Complete Part I
5	Supp. E-3		Complete, if applicable
6	E	29	Complete Part II, lines 2, 4 and 5; complete lines 21 through 24, as appropriate
7	Title XVIII Supp. E-4 or Supp. E-4-1		Complete the appropriate part or parts, if applicable
8	E	30	Complete Part III, line 1 and lines 3 through 6
9	E-2	32	Complete entire worksheet

140 PRINCIPLES OF REIMBURSEMENT IN HEALTH CARE

Step No.	Worksheet	Page(s)	
10	E	30	Complete Part III, lines 7 through 17
11	E-1	31	Complete lines 1 through 4
12	E	30	Complete Part III, lines 18 and 19
13	E-5	33	Complete Part I; complete Part II, line 2 and line 4; complete line 16 or 17, as appropriate
14	Titles V & XIX Supp. E-4 or Supp. E-4-1		Complete the appropriate part or parts, if applicable
15	E-5	34	Complete Part III, line 1 and lines 3 through 11, as appropriate
16	G	35	Providers maintaining fund type accounting records should complete the worksheet in its entirety Providers not maintaining fund type accounting records should complete the "General Fund" columns only.
17	G-1	36	Providers maintaining fund type accounting records should complete the worksheet in its entirety. Providers not maintaining fund type accounting records should complete the "General Fund" columns only.
18	G-2	37	Complete entire worksheet
19	G-3	38	Complete entire worksheet

302(Cont.)   FORM HCFA-2552   8-80

Step No.	Worksheet	Page(s)	
20	Worksheet Checklist	1	Complete entire worksheet
21		2	Complete Certification Statement

PART VI - Calculation of Reimbursement Settlement

Public Providers Rendering Services Free of Charge or at a Nominal Charge:

1	E	28	Complete Part I
2	D-8	27	Complete as appropriate
3	Supp. E-3		Complete, if applicable
4	Title XVIII Supp. E-4-1		Complete Part I and/or Part II, if applicable
5	E	30	Complete Part III, lines 1, 3, 4 and 6
6	E-2	32	Complete entire worksheet
7	E	30	Complete Part III, lines 7 through 10 and lines 13 through 17, as applicable
8	E-1	31	Complete lines 1 through 4
9	E	30	Complete Part III, lines 18 and 19
10	E-5	33	Complete Part I
11	Titles V & XIX Supp. E-4-1		Complete Part I and/or Part II, if applicable
12	E-5	34	Complete Part III, lines 1, 3, 5 and 7 through 11
13	G	35	Complete entire worksheet
14	G-1	36	Complete entire worksheet
15	G-2	37	Complete entire worksheet
16	G-3	38	Complete entire worksheet

3-14   Rev. 10

Step No.	Worksheet	Page(s)	
17	Worksheet Checklist	1	Complete entire worksheet
18		2	Complete Certification Statement

303. WORKSHEET CHECKLIST
The purpose of this Worksheet Checklist is to identify each worksheet that is being completed or not being completed as a part of this cost report. Worksheets which are not completed because they are not applicable to the provider are not required to be submitted as a part of this cost report.

Columns 1 through 3 - Check the appropriate column for each worksheet. When column 2 is checked, provide the information at the bottom of this worksheet. When column 3 is checked, inclusion of a blank worksheet is not required.

Statistical Data

304. HOSPITAL, HOSPITAL-SKILLED NURSING FACILITY COMPLEX AND SKILLED NURSING FACILITY STATISTICAL DATA

304.1 Part I - General.--

ITEM 1. NAMES AND ADDRESSES, PROVIDER NUMBERS AND DATES CERTIFIED. Enter on the appropriate lines the names and addresses, provider or identification numbers and certification dates of the facility and its various components, if any. The following definitions apply when completing these cost reporting forms.

HOSPITAL--An institution meeting the requirements of section 1861(e) of the "Health Insurance for the Aged and Disabled Act" and participating in the Medicare program, or a Federally controlled institution approved by the Secretary.

SUBPROVIDER--A general hospital which has been issued subprovider identification numbers because it offers clearly different types of service, e.g., short-term acute and long-term tuberculosis. See PRM, Part I, chapter 23, for a complete explanation of separate cost entities in multiple facility hospitals.

SKILLED NURSING FACILITY--An institution meeting the requirements of section 1861(j) of the "Health Insurance for the Aged and Disabled Act" and participating in the Medicare program, or a Federally controlled institution approved by the Secretary.

HOSPITAL-BASED SKILLED NURSING FACILITY--A distinct part and separately certified component of a hospital where skilled nursing and related services are provided.

HOME HEALTH AGENCY--An institution meeting the requirements of section 1861(o) of the "Health Insurance for the Aged and Disabled Act" and participating in the Medicare program, or a Federally controlled institution approved by the Secretary. The remainder of the statistical data for a provider-based home health agency should be entered on form HCFA-1728A.

SPECIAL PROVIDER-CONTROLLED FACILITY--A separate cost entity controlled and/or owned by one provider or jointly by more than one provider. This entity usually has its own administration, staff, building, location and financial autonomy. Examples include a provider-controlled comprehensive health center and a patient service facility financed and operated by two or more providers on a shared-cost basis. The services rendered are under the control of the provider(s) and are services usually covered for Medicare reimbursement by title XVIII statutory or regulatory provisions. A special provider-controlled facility could not participate in the Medicare program in the absence of the provider or providers to which it is related.

ITEM 2. COST REPORTING PERIOD.
Enter the inclusive dates covered by this cost report. Generally, a cost reporting period consists of 12 consecutive calendar months or 13 four-week periods with an additional day (two in a leap year) added to the last week or period to make it coincide with the end of the calendar year or month. See PRM, Part I, chapter 24, for situations where a short period cost report may be filed.

Cost reports are due on or before the last day of the third month following the close of the provider's accounting (Medicare cost reporting) period.

A 30-day extension of the due date of a cost report may, for good cause, be granted by the intermediary after first obtaining approval of the Health Care Financing Administration.

The final cost report of a provider which voluntarily or involuntarily ceases to participate in the health insurance program is due no later than 45 days following the effective date of the termination of the provider agreement including termination of the provider agreement as a result of a change of ownership. There are no provisions for an extension of the cost report due date with respect to providers which cease to participate in the program.

ITEM 3. TYPE OF CONTROL.
Indicate the type of ownership or auspices under which the institution is conducted.

Medicare Regulations Regarding Hospital Accounting Techniques

The following Medicare instructions apply, at this writing, to the use of hospital accounting techniques, as discussed in Chapter 4. Relevant worksheets, identified by exhibit number from the list of worksheets in Appendix F, follow the instructions. Accounting techniques are applied on Medicare Worksheet A through Worksheet A-8-1.

If the scope of review covers all patients, all allowable costs
should be reclassified in column 4 to Administrative and General
Expense (line 5). If the scope of the review covers only
Medicare patients or Medicare, title V and title XIX patients,
(1) in column 4, reclassify to Administrative and General Expense
all allowable costs other than physicians' compensation and
(2) deduct in column 6, the compensation paid to the physicians
for their personal services on the utilization review committee.
When a hospital-based skilled nursing facility is not under PSRO
review, direct PSRO review costs must not be included with
utilization review costs for skilled nursing facilities on this
line. (See PRM, Part I, chapter 21, for further details.)

Line 70 - PSRO - Federal or Combined--Enter on this line the total
amount of direct review costs for hospitals which perform delegated acute care and/or long term care PSRO review for Federal
patients only (if there are no utilization review activities for
non-Federal patients) or for all patients if the same type and
intensity of review is applied to Federal and non-Federal patients.
When a hospital-based skilled nursing facility is not under PSRO
review, direct PSRO review costs must not be included with
utilization review costs for skilled nursing facilities on line 69.
(See PRM, Part I, 1975 Amendments, Supplemental 1.)

Where the amounts entered on Worksheet A, column 6, differ from
the entries on form HCFA-153, a supporting worksheet reconciling
the costs must be included in this cost report.

Line 71 - PSRO - Non-Federal--Enter on this line the total amount
of direct PSRO review costs attributable to non-Federal patients
only. This line is used only when the review activities for
non-Federal patients are different in type and intensity from
those applied to Federal patients. When a hospital-based skilled
nursing facility is not under PSRO review, direct PSRO review
costs must not be included with utilization review costs for
skilled nursing facilities on line 69. (See PRM, Part I, 1975
Amendments, Supplemental 1.)

Where the amounts entered on Worksheet A, column 6, differ from
the entries on form HCFA-153, a supporting worksheet reconciling
the costs must be included in this cost report.

Lines 75 through 79--Providers will use these lines to record the
costs applicable to nonreimbursable cost centers to which general
service center costs apply. However, where the expense (direct and
all applicable overhead) attributable to any nonallowable cost area
is so insignificant as not to warrant establishment of a nonreimbursable cost center and the sum total of all such expenses is so
insignificant as not to warrant establishment of a composite
nonreimbursable cost center, these expenses may be adjusted on
Worksheet A-8. (See PRM, Part I, chapter 23.)

Line 77 - Physicians' Private Offices--A nonreimbursable cost
center must be established to accumulate the cost incurred by the
provider for services related to the physicians' private practice.
Examples of such costs are depreciation costs for the space
occupied, movable equipment used by the physicians' offices,
administrative services, medical records, housekeeping, maintenance and repairs, operation of plant, drugs, medical supplies,
nursing service, etc.

This nonreimbursable cost center should not include costs
applicable to services rendered to hospital patients by hospital
based physicians. Such costs may be properly includable in
hospital costs.

Line 79--Providers will use this line to record the cost applicable
to any nonreimbursable cost center not provided for on this worksheet. For example, where a determination has been made that a
provider furnishes luxury items or services, a nonreimbursable
cost center entitled "Luxury Routine Accommodations" must be
established to accumulate the excess cost of the luxury items.
(See PRM, Part I, chapter 21, for further details.)

Line 79 should be appropriately labeled to indicate the purpose
for which it is being used. If additional space is needed, any
available line below line 74 may be used.

308. WORKSHEET A-1 - RECLASSIFICATION AFFECTING ADMINISTRATIVE
      AND GENERAL EXPENSES
This worksheet provides for the reclassification of certain amounts
to effect proper cost allocation under cost finding. Certain
expenses pertaining to buildings and fixtures and movable equipment must be allocated or directly assigned on the same basis as
the respective depreciation expenses; such as, insurance on
buildings and fixtures and movable equipment, rent on buildings
and fixtures and movable equipment, interest on funds borrowed
to purchase buildings and fixtures and movable equipment, personal
property taxes, and real property taxes. However, interest on
funds borrowed for operating expense must be allocated with
administrative and general expenses.

Providers may have changed some of these amounts to the proper
cost center before the end of the accounting period. THEREFORE,
WORKSHEET A-1 SHOULD BE COMPLETED ONLY TO THE EXTENT THAT.EXPENSES
HAVE BEEN INCLUDED IN COST CENTERS THAT WOULD DIFFER FROM THE
RESULT THAT WOULD BE OBTAINED USING THE INSTRUCTION OF THE PRECEDING
PARAGRAPH.

Lines 2 through 12--Enter in column 3, lines 2 through 12, the
Employee Health and Welfare Expenses included in the Administrative
and General cost center (Worksheet A, column 3, line 5).

Line 13--Enter on this line, in columns 3 and 4, the total Employee Health and Welfare Expense included in the Administrative and General cost center.

Line 14--Enter in the appropriate columns on line 14, the insurance expense included in the Administrative and General cost center on Worksheet A, column 3, line 5, which is applicable to buildings and fixtures and movable equipment.

Line 15--Enter in the appropriate columns on line 15, any interest expense included in Worksheet A, column 3, line 68, which is applicable to funds borrowed for administrative and general purposes (operating expenses, etc.) or for the purchase of buildings and fixtures or movable equipment.

Line 16--Enter in the appropriate columns on line 16, rent expenses included in the Administrative and General cost center on Worksheet A, column 3, line 5, which is applicable to the rental of buildings and fixtures and to movable equipment from other than related organizations. See instructions for Worksheet A-8-1 for treatment of rental expense with respect to related organizations.

Line 17--Enter in the appropriate columns, any taxes (real property taxes and/or personal property taxes) included in the Administrative and General cost center on Worksheet A, column 3, line 5.

Line 18--This line pertains only to a skilled nursing facility or the hospital-based skilled nursing facility. If the scope of the utilization review covers the entire patient population, enter on line 18, columns 4 and 6, the total allowable utilization review costs included on Worksheet A, column 3, line 69. However, where the scope of the utilization review in the skilled nursing facility covers only Medicare patients or Medicare, title V and title XIX patients, only the allowable utilization review costs included on Worksheet A, column 3, line 69, other than the compensation of physicians for their personal services on utilization review committees should be entered on line 18, columns 4 and 6.

The appropriate adjustment for physicians' compensation should be made on Worksheet A-8, column 2, line 60. For further explanations concerning utilization review in skilled nursing facilities, see PRM, Part I, chapter 21.

Line 19--Enter the column totals on line 19 and transfer such amounts to the appropriate lines on Worksheet A, column 4.

310. WORKSHEET A-2 - RECLASSIFICATION OF DIETARY EXPENSE

The purpose of this worksheet is to reclassify the expense included
in the Dietary cost center applicable to the cafeteria, nursery
and to any other cost centers such as gift, coffee shop and
canteen and to apportion any unidentified dietary costs to the
appropriate cost centers.

A provider is prohibited from using this worksheet if it makes a
completely separate and distinct accounting for the costs of the
cafeteria, nursery and other appropriate cost centers because
such cost centers are organizationally independent of the dietary
inpatient food service.

Also, a provider which has developed the accounting capability to
distribute dietary costs on the basis of weighted meals is not
required to submit this worksheet, but may submit its own worksheet for reclassifying dietary expense. The substitute worksheet
must show both the statistical data used as the basis for determining weighted meals and the actual distribution of the dietary
costs.

The use of any alternative method for reclassifying dietary
expense is subject to intermediary approval. Once an
alternative method is approved by the intermediary, the provider
may not revert to the use of Worksheet A-2 for the reclassification
of dietary expense.

PART I - RECLASSIFICATION OF EXPENSES

Column 1--Enter on lines 3 through 5, as appropriate, the costs
shown on Worksheet A, column 3. These amounts constitute the
costs identified with the cafeteria, nursery, etc., as recorded
in the provider's accounting records.

Column 2--Enter on line 1 the total dietary expense from
Worksheet A, column 3, line 10. Enter on lines 2 through 5 the
amounts included in the dietary expense on line 1, which are
specifically identifiable in the accounting records, or by
analysis as being incurred for the respective cost centers. The
total of these identified expenses is entered on line 6. The
total unidentified dietary expenses (line 1 minus line 6) is
entered on line 7 and will be allocated in columns 4 and 5.

Column 3--On each line enter the sum of columns 1 and 2. The
totals entered in column 3 represent the basis upon which the
unidentified expenses will be allocated.

Column 4--Enter the ratios as indicated on the worksheet. These
ratios will be used to allocate the total unidentified expenses
(column 2, line 7) and are computed by dividing the identified

expenses (column 3, lines 2, 3, 4 and 5, respectively) by the total
identified dietary expenses (column 3, line 6).

PART II - TRANSFER OF RECLASSIFIED EXPENSES
This part provides for the transfer to Worksheet A, column 4, of
the reclassified expenses which were included in the Dietary cost
center, as determined in Part I.

312. WORKSHEET A-3 - RECLASSIFICATION OF CENTRAL SERVICES AND
      SUPPLY
This worksheet provides for reclassifying the direct expenses
included in the Central Services and Supply cost center, but
which are directly applicable to other cost centers, such as
Intern-Resident Services, Intravenous Therapy, Oxygen (Inhalation)
Therapy, etc. Additional space is provided for the reclassification needed to effect proper cost allocation of other expenses
included therein.

314. WORKSHEET A-4 - RECLASSIFICATION OF LABORATORY EXPENSE
This worksheet provides for reclassifying the direct expenses
included in the Laboratory cost center, but which are directly
applicable to other cost centers, such as Whole Blood and Packed
Red Blood Cells, Electrocardiology, etc. Additional space is
provided for the reclassification needed to effect proper cost
allocation of other expenses.

316. WORKSHEET A-5 - RECLASSIFICATION OF RADIOLOGY - DIAGNOSTIC
This worksheet provides for reclassifying the direct expenses
included in the Radiology-Diagnostic cost center, but which are
directly applicable to other cost centers, such as Radiology-
Therapeutic, Radioisotope, Electrocardiology, etc. Additional
space is provided for the reclassification needed to effect
proper cost allocation of other expenses.

318. WORKSHEET A-6 - RECLASSIFICATIONS - OTHER
This worksheet provides for the reclassification of expenses in
addition to those provided for on Worksheets A-1 through A-5.

The following are some examples of costs which should be
reclassified on this worksheet.

        1. Where a provider purchases services (e.g., physical
therapy) under arrangements for Medicare patients, but does not
purchase such services under arrangements for non-Medicare
patients, the providers' books will reflect only the cost of the
Medicare services. However, if the provider does not use the
"grossing up" technique for purposes of allocating overhead, and
if the provider incurs related direct costs applicable to all
patients, Medicare and non-Medicare (e.g., paramedics or aides
who assist a physical therapist in performing physical therapy
services) such related costs should be reclassified on

Worksheet A-6 from the ancillary service cost center and be allocated as part of administrative and general expense. (See PRM, Part I, chapter 23.)

2. Rental expense on movable equipment which was charged directly to the appropriate cost center or cost centers must be reclassified on this worksheet to the Depreciation-Movable Equipment cost center unless the provider has identified and charged all depreciation on movable equipment to the appropriate cost centers.

3. The provisions on guaranteed standby fees as explained in PRM, Part I, chapter 21, apply when the hospital guarantees emergency room physicians a minimum level of compensation for being on a standby basis to handle emergencies. When charges for the physician services fall short of the guaranteed amount, the difference paid by the hospital is recognized as a provider cost. These provisions are applicable whether the provider or the physician bills for physician services.

The unmet guarantee amount recognized as a hospital cost for Medicare reimbursement purposes is determined as follows:

a. Reduce the guarantee by that portion of the physician compensation attributable to administrative and supervisory duties. The physician compensation attributable to administrative and supervisory duties should be reclassified where necessary to the appropriate cost centers.

b. Determine the total billing value of services provided by the physicians. This amount would include the actual emergency room billings by the physicians as well as the assigned value of services rendered for which these physicians are prohibited from charging under the terms of their contract.

c. Standby cost is determined by subtracting the billing value of services (see b above) from the adjusted guarantee (see a above).

The Medicare portion of this unmet guarantee amount (standby cost) would be reimbursed as reasonable cost under the Medicare program. The unmet guarantee is distributed to the appropriate cost centers (emergency, general routine care, etc.) in the same ratio that the physician charges attributable to each of the cost centers bears to the total billing value of physician services.

Transfer the net amount of the reclassification of the unmet guarantee expenses attributable to each cost center to the appropriate line on Worksheet A, column 4.

152   PRINCIPLES OF REIMBURSEMENT IN HEALTH CARE

Note, any income (i.e., gross physician charges less bad debts and contractual allowances) realized by the hospital in excess of its payments to the physician must be used as an offset against hospital costs. Accordingly, such income must be offset against the appropriate cost center in the same ratio that the standby cost would have been distributed.

320.   WORKSHEET A-7 - LIMITATION ON FEDERAL PARTICIPATION FOR CAPITAL EXPENDITURES QUESTIONNAIRE

Line 1--The analysis of changes in capital asset balances during the cost reporting period must be completed by all hospitals, skilled nursing facilities and hospital-skilled nursing facility complexes. The amount to be entered should not be reduced by any accumulated depreciation reserves.

Columns 1 and 6--Enter the balance recorded in the provider's books of account at the beginning of the provider's cost reporting period (column 1) and at the end of the provider's cost reporting period (column 6).

Columns 2 through 4--Enter the cost of capital assets acquired by purchase (including assets transferred from another provider, noncertified health care unit or nonhealth care unit) in column 2, and the fair market value at date acquired of donated assets in column 3. Enter the sum of columns 2 and 3 in column 4.

Column 5--Enter the cost or rther approved basis of all capital assets sold, traded, transferred to another provider, a noncertified health care unit or nonhealth care unit, retired or disposed of in any other manner during the provider's cost reporting period.

The sum of columns 1 and 4 minus column 5 should equal column 6.

Line 2--A "Capital Expenditure" which is subject to the provisions of section 1122 of the Social Security Act is an expenditure for plant and equipment that is not properly chargeable as an expense of operation and maintenance and (1) exceeds $100,000 or (2) changes the bed capacity of the facility or (3) substantially changes the services of the facility. See PRM, Part I, chapter 24, for further explanation.

LINES 3 AND 4 WILL NOT BE COMPLETED IF THE ANSWER TO LINE 2 IS "NO."

Line 3--The data requested must be provided for each capital expenditure (as defined in PRM, Part I, chapter 24) made by or on behalf of the provider during the period to which this cost report applies and (1) subsequent to December 31, 1972, or (2) the effective date of the agreement between the State and the Secretary, whichever is later.

Column 1--Use the following symbols to indicate how the asset was acquired: "A" by purchase on the open market; "B" by donation or transfer; and "C" by lease or comparable arrangement.

Column 2--Enter the date on which the obligation for the capital expenditure was incurred by or on behalf of the provider, or in the case of donated assets, the date the capital expenditure was acquired by the provider.

Column 3--The cost of the capital expenditure includes the cost of studies, surveys, designs, plans, working drawings, specifications and other activities essential to the acquisition, improvement, modernization, expansion or replacement of the land, plant, buildings and equipment. Also, included are expenditures directly or indirectly related to capital expenditures, including expenses with respect to grading, paving, broker commissions, taxes assessed during the construction period and costs involved in demolishing or razing structures on land.

Columns 4 through 9--All expenses included on Worksheet A, column 5, related to capital expenditures made in this cost reporting period must be included in columns 4, 5, 6 and 8, as appropriate.

The type of expense included in column 8 should be described in column 7.

The sum of the expenses entered in columns 4, 5, 6 and 8 must equal the amount entered in column 9.

Line 4--

Column 1--Enter the date on which the written notice of intention for each capital expenditure by or on behalf of the provider was submitted to the Designated Planning Agency.

IF THE WRITTEN NOTICE SUBMITTED TO THE DESIGNATED PLANNING AGENCY IS STILL PENDING, DO NOT COMPLETE COLUMNS 2 THROUGH 5.

Column 2--Enter the date of notification of approval by the Designated Planning Agency for each capital expenditure made by or on behalf of the provider.

IF A CAPITAL EXPENDITURE WAS APPROVED, COLUMNS 3 THROUGH 5 SHOULD NOT BE COMPLETED.

Column 3--Enter in column 3 the date the notice of disapproval of the capital expenditure was received from the Designated Planning Agency.

NOTE: Where the Designated Planning Agency determines a capital expenditure is inconsistent with the State or local

planning requirements, the provider must make an adjustment
on Worksheet A-8, line 19, to exclude any expenses included
on Worksheet A, column 5, related to the disapproved
capital expenditures.

Columns 4 and 5--Complete columns 4 and 5 only if the Designated
Planning Agency's decision has been appealed. If the decision
has been appealed, show the date and status of appeal in
columns 4 and 5, respectively.

322. WORKSHEET A-8 - ADJUSTMENTS TO EXPENSES
This worksheet consists of two pages and provides for the
adjustments to the expenses listed on Worksheet A, column 5.
These adjustments, which are required under the Medicare Principles
of Reimbursement, are to be made on the basis of "cost," or
"amount received." Enter the total "amount received" (revenue)
only if the cost (including direct cost and all applicable overhead) cannot be determined; but, if the total direct and indirect
cost can be determined, enter the "cost." Once an adjustment
to an expense is made on the basis of "cost," the provider may
not in future cost reporting periods determine the required
adjustment to the expense on the basis of "revenue." The
following symbols are to be entered in column 1 to indicate the
basis for adjustment: "A" for cost; and "B" for amount received.
Line descriptions indicate the more common activities which
affect allowable costs, or result in costs incurred for reasons
other than patient care and, thus, require adjustments.

Types of items to be entered on Worksheet A-8 are (1) those
needed to adjust expenses to reflect actual expenses incurred;
(2) those items which constitute recovery of expenses through
sales, charges, fees, grants, gifts, etc.; (3) those items needed
to adjust expenses in accordance with the Medicare Principles of
Reimbursement; and (4) those items which are provided for
separately in the cost apportionment process.

Where an adjustment to an expense affects more than one cost
center, the provider should record the adjustment to each cost
center on a separate line on Worksheet A-8.

LINE DESCRIPTIONS

Line 1 - Investment Income on Commingled Restricted and Unrestricted
Funds--Investment income on restricted and unrestricted funds
which are commingled with other funds must be applied together
against, but should not exceed, the total interest expense
included in allowable costs. (See PRM, Part I, chapter 2.)

The investment income on restricted and unrestricted funds which
are commingled with other funds should be applied against the
Administrative and General, the Depreciation-Buildings and

322(Cont.)   FORM HCFA-2552   8-80

Fixtures, the Depreciation-Movable Equipment and any other
appropriate cost centers on the basis of the ratio that interest
expense charged to each cost center bears to the total interest
expense charged to all of the provider's cost centers.

Line 8 - Remuneration Applicable to Provider-Based Radiologists
for Professional Services

Line 9 - Remuneration Applicable to Provider-Based Pathologists
for Professional Services

Line 10 - Remuneration Applicable to Provider-Based Anesthesiologists
for Professional Services

Line 11 - Remuneration Applicable to Provider-Based Cardiologists
for Professional Services

Line 12 - Remuneration Applicable to Provider--Based Neurologists
for Professional Services--Enter on the appropriate line, the
total amount of wages, salaries and fees, including all applicable
fringe benefits, paid to provider-based physicians for personal
patient care services rendered. Enter all such amounts whether
or not the provider is using combined billing. Amounts paid to
provider-based physicians for general hospital services, rendered
are not to be included in these adjustments. (See PRM, Part I,
chapter 21.)

Lines 13-16, 30, 31, 45-57 and 63--Enter on these lines any
additional adjustments which are required under the Medicare
Principles of Reimbursement. The lines should be appropriately
labeled to indicate the nature of the required adjustments.

An example of an adjustment which would be entered on these
lines is the "grossing up" of costs in accordance with provisions
of the PRM, Part I, chapter 23, and as explained below.

Where a provider furnishes ancillary services to health care
program patients under arrangements with others, but simply
arranges for such services for nonhealth care program patients
and does not pay the nonhealth care program portion of such
services, its books will reflect only the cost of the health care
program portion. Therefore, allocation of indirect costs to a
cost center which includes only the cost of the health care
program portion would result in excessive assignment of indirect
costs to the health care programs. Since services were also
arranged for the nonhealth care program patients, part of the
overhead costs should be allocated to those groups.

In the foregoing situation, no indirect costs may be allocated
to the cost center unless the intermediary determines that the

provider is able to "gross up" both the costs and the charges for
services to nonhealth care program patients so that both costs
and charges for services to nonhealth care program patients are
recorded as if the provider had provided such services directly.
See the instructions for Worksheet C with respect to "grossing
up" of the provider's charges.

Line 17 - Home Office Costs--Enter on this line allowable home
office costs which have been allocated to the provider. Additional lines should be used to the extent that various provider
cost centers are affected. (See PRM, Part I, chapter 21.)

Line 20 - Adjustment Resulting From Transactions with Related
Organizations--The amount to be entered on this line is obtained
from Worksheet A-8-1, Part B, column 6, line 10. Note that
Worksheet A-8-1, Part B, lines 1-9, represent the detail of the
various cost centers to be adjusted on Worksheet A.

Line 29 - Income from Imposition of Interest, Finance or Penalty
Charges--Enter on this line the cash received from imposition
of interest, finance or penalty charges on overdue receivables.
This income must be used to offset the allowable administrative
and general costs. See PRM, Part I, chapter 21.

Line 32--Enter on this line the sum of lines 1 through 31 and
carry forward this subtotal to page 11, line 33.

Line 34 - Adjustment for Physical Therapy Costs in Excess of
Limitation--The amount to be entered on this line is obtained
from Supplemental Worksheet A-8-3, line 42.

Definitions Applicable to Lines 35 through 41

> Malpractice Premiums and/or Self-Insurance
> Fund Contributions (line 35)--When a
> provider has combined coverage for
> malpractice and comprehensive general
> liability, the provider must obtain from
> the commercial insurance company or the
> fiduciary for the self-insurance fund
> an actuarial determination of the
> portion of the insurance premium or
> the self-insurance fund contribution
> (including related expenses - PRM
> Part I, section 2162.8) applicable to
> malpractice.
>
> Allowable Paid Malpractice Losses--
> Titles V, XVIII and XIX (lines 36,
> 38 and 40.--Allowable paid malpractice

322(Cont.)   FORM HCFA-2552   8-80

losses are the actual amounts paid to
the claimant by the provider. These
include amounts paid for uninsured
malpractice losses through allowable
deductible or coinsurance provisions
(PRM, Part I, section 2162.5), as a
result of a loss in excess of reasonable
coverage limits (PRM, Part I, section
2162.6), or by a governmental provider
(PRM, Part I, section 2162.14). "Accrued"
or "estimated" malpractice losses are
not allowable.

A malpractice loss arises from an
incident resulting from medical practices and procedures which caused
injuries or damages to an individual who
is a patient of a provider. A patient is
further defined to include any individual
perambulating or being transported on
provider premises in the course of seeking
specific inpatient or outpatient services
or as a result of receiving such services.
Incidents causing injuries or damages to
patients that would be classified as
malpractice include, but are not limited
to:

    Surgical error;
    Misdiagnosis of an illness or injury;
    Incorrect treatment or medication.

Incidents involving nonpatients of the
provider or incidents not resulting from
medical practices and procedures are not
recognized as malpractice incidents.

An allowable paid malpractice loss is
classified as title V, XVIII or XIX on the
basis of the patient's coverage at the time
the malpractice incident occurs. For
example, when a malpractice incident occurs
on a day when the patient is receiving
provider services covered under Medicare
Part A or Part B, the malpractice loss is
classified as a title XVIII malpractice loss.

If a provider chooses not to file a
claim for a malpractice loss that is
covered by insurance, the loss and any
related direct expenses are unallowable.

Allowable Related Direct Expenses--
Titles V, XVIII and XIX (lines 37, 39
and 41).--Costs related directly to
allowable paid malpractice losses (i.e.,
lines 36, 38 and 40) are 100 percent
directly assigned to titles V, XVIII
or XIX. These costs include incurred
amounts for claims processing, legal
fees, court proceedings, witness
expenses and interest on necessary and
proper loans made for the sole purpose
of paying direct assigned losses.

Line 35 - Malpractice Premiums and/or Self-Insurance Fund
Contributions--Enter the amount of malpractice insurance premiums
and/or self-insurance fund contributions incurred. A separate
apportionment of these costs to the Federal health care programs
will be completed on Worksheet D-8.

NOTE: Where the health care complex can specifically identify
         the amount of malpractice premiums and/or fund
         contributions for each component of the health care
         complex, a separate adjustment for each component of
         the health care complex must be shown and identified.

Lines 36-41--Enter on these lines amounts paid for allowable
uninsured malpractice losses as a result of the application of
deductible or coinsurance provisions of a purchased insurance
policy or a funded self-insurance program within the guidelines
established in the PRM, Part I, chapter 21, or as a result of an
award in excess of reasonable coverage limits, or as a
governmental provider. Such losses and related direct costs
must be identified for titles V, XVIII and XIX, excluding such
losses and related direct costs for the home health agency.

Line 42--Enter on this line the amounts paid for home health agency allowable uninsured malpractice losses (Federal and non-Federal) as a result of the application of deductible or coinsurance provisions of a purchased insurance policy or a funded self-insurance program within the guidelines established in the PRM, Part I, chapter 21, or a result of an award in excess of reasonable coverage limits, or as a governmental provider. Such losses and related direct costs must be identified for the home health agency only.

Also, include on this line the amount of malpractice premiums and/or fund contributions (Federal and non-Federal) specifically identified to the home health agency. (See instructions to line 35.)

Line 43--Enter on this line any nonallowable malpractice insurance premiums and/or self-insurance fund contributions. Also, enter all nonallowable uninsured malpractice losses and the related direct costs for Federal patients. In addition, enter uninsured malpractice losses and the related direct costs for non-Federal patients excluding such losses and related direct costs for the home health agency.

NOTE: The sum of lines 35 through 43 must equal the amount on Worksheet A, column 5, line 67.

Line 45 - PSRO Costs (Federal or Combined)--Enter the total amount of direct review costs on Worksheet A, column 5, line 70.

Line 46 - PSRO Costs (Non-Federal Only)--Enter the total amount of direct review costs on Worksheet A, column 5, line 71.

Line 58--Enter on this line the sum of lines 33 through 57.

Line 59 - Grants, Gifts and Income Designated by Donor for Specific Expenses--Enter on line 59, any grants, gifts or endowment income designated by a donor for paying specific operating costs which are included on Worksheet A, column 5. Also, enter any carry-over of the excess of grants, gifts or endowment income over the specific operating costs incurred in a prior cost reporting period.

If the grant, gift or endowment income has been designated to pay for a specific operating expense within a cost center, the amount of such income to be entered on line 59 should not exceed the total of the specific operating expense stipulated in the restriction established by the donor. Any excess of the income over the direct costs should be carried over to the subsequent cost reporting year.

On the other hand, if the grant, gift or endowment income has been designated to pay for the operating costs of an entire cost center, the provider must use all such income as an offset even though it exceeds the specific direct operating costs shown on Worksheet A, column 5. Any excess of the income over the direct cost should be shown in parentheses (   ).

See the instructions for Worksheet B concerning the treatment of any such excess with respect to cost finding and the possible carryover to the subsequent cost reporting period.

NOTE: Do not include on this line any Federal research grants or any other grants, gifts or endowment income pertaining to any nonreimbursable cost centers which are included on Worksheet B.

Line 60 - Utilization Review - Physicians' Compensation--This line pertains to the skilled nursing facility and the hospital based skilled nursing facility only. When the utilization review covers only Medicare patients or Medicare, title V and title XIX patients, the reasonable compensation paid to the physicians for their services on utilization review committees is to be allocated 100 percent to the health care programs. The amount attributable to Medicare patients will be included on Worksheet E, Part I, column 7, line 5 (Computation of Net Cost of Covered Services). All other allowable costs applicable to utilization review which covers only health care program patients are to be apportioned among all users of the skilled nursing facility or hospital-based skilled nursing facility. Such other costs should have been reclassified on Worksheet A-1, line 18. Enter on this line the physicians' compensation for services on utilization review committees which cover only health care program patients in the skilled nursing facility or hospital-based skilled nursing facility. The amount entered should equal the amount shown on Worksheet A, column 5, line 69.

Line 61 - Depreciation - Buildings and Fixtures and Line 62 - Depreciation - Movable Equipment--Where depreciation expense computed in accordance with the Medicare Principles of Reimbursement differs from depreciation expenses per the provider's books, enter the difference on lines 61 and/or 52. (See PRM, Part I, chapter 1.)

Line 64--Enter on this line the amount on line 58 plus or minus the sum of lines 59 through 63. TRANSFER THE AMOUNTS IN COLUMN 2 TO WORKSHEET A, COLUMN 6.

324. WORKSHEET A-8-1 - STATEMENT OF COSTS OF SERVICES FROM RELATED ORGANIZATIONS

This worksheet provides for the computation of any needed adjustments to costs applicable to services, facilities and supplies furnished to the provider by organizations related to the provider by common ownership or control. In addition, certain information concerning the related organizations with which the provider has transacted business should be shown. (See PRM, Part I, chapter 10.)

PART A must be completed by all providers. If the answer to
Part A is "Yes," Parts B and C must also be completed.

PART B - Costs applicable to services, facilities and supplies
furnished to the provider by organizations related to the provider
by common ownership or control are includable in the allowable
cost of the provider at the cost to the related organizations.
However, such cost must not exceed the amount a prudent and
cost-conscious buyer would pay for comparable services, facilities
or supplies that could be purchased elsewhere.

PART C - This part is used to show the interrelationship of the
provider to organizations furnishing services, facilities or
supplies to the provider. The requested data relative to all
individuals, partnerships, corporations or other organizations
having either a related interest to the provider, a common
ownership of the provider, or control over the provider as defined
in PRM, Part I, chapter 10, must be shown in columns 1 through 6,
as appropriate.

Only those columns which are pertinent to the type of relationship
which exists should be completed.

Column 1--Enter the appropriate symbol which describes the
interrelationship of the provider to the related organization.

Column 2--If the symbol A, D, E, F or G is entered in column 1,
enter the name of the related individual in column 2.

Column 3--If the individual in column 2 or the organization in
column 4 has a financial interest in the provider, enter in this
column the percent of ownership in the provider.

Column 4--Enter in this column the name of the related corporation,
partnership or other organization.

Column 5--If the individual in column 2 or the provider has a
financial interest in the related organization, enter in this
column the percent of ownership in such organization.

Column 6--Enter in this column the type of business in which the
related organization engages (e.g., medical drugs and/or supplies,
laundry and linen service).

326. WORKSHEET A-8-2 - DEPRECIATION
This worksheet provides for furnishing certain information
concerning depreciation. All items should be completed. (See
PRM, Part I, chapter 1.)

Exhibit 5

HOSPITAL, SKILLED NURSING FACILITY AND HEALTH CARE COMPLEX STATISTICAL DATA	PROVIDER NO.:	PERIOD: FROM_____ TO_____

PART VI—HOME HEALTH AGENCY STATISTICS

		Title XVIII		Other		TOTAL	
		Visits	Patients	Visits	Patients	Visits	Patients
1	Home Health Agency Visits	1	2	3	4	5	6
	a. Skilled Nursing						
	b. Physical Therapy						
	c. Speech Pathology						
	d. Occupational Therapy						
	e. Medical Social Service						
	f. Home Health Aide						
	g. All Other Services						
	h. Total Visits (Sum of lines 1a–1g)						
	i. Unduplicated Census Count						
	j. Home Health Aide Hours						

2 Home Health Agency—Number of Employees (Full Time Equivalent)

	Enter the number of hours IN YOUR NORMAL WORK WEEK _____	STAFF	CONTRACT	TOTAL
		1	2	3
a. Administrator & Assistant Administrators				
b. Directors & Assistant Directors				
c. Other Administrative Personnel				
d. Direct Nursing Service				
e. Nursing Supervisor				
f. Physical Therapy Service				
g. Physical Therapy Supervisor				
h. Speech Pathology Service				
i. Speech Pathology Supervisor				
j. Occupational Therapy Service				
k. Occupational Therapy Supervisor				
l. Medical Social Service				
m. Medical Social Service Supervisor				
n. Home Health Aide				
o. Home Health Aide Supervisor				
p.				
q.				

PART VII—RENAL DIALYSIS DEPARTMENT STATISTICS

1 Renal Dialysis Statistics

Type of Physician Reimbursement Method	☐ Initial ☐ Alternative		Date for Election for Alternative Method _____	
	OUTPATIENT		TRAINING	
	Hemodialysis	Peritoneal Dialysis	Hemodialysis	Peritoneal Dialysis
	1	2	3	4
a. Number of Treatments Not Billed to Medicare & Furnished Directly				
b. Number of Treatments Not Billed to Medicare & Furnished Under Arrangements				
c. Average times per week patient receives dialysis				
d. Number of days in an average week for patient dialysis treatments				
e. Average time of patient dialysis treatment including set up time				
f. Number of machines regularly available for use				
g. Number of standby machines				
h. Machine time used in typical week during regular reporting period per shift				

i. Type of dialyzers used. If dialyzers are reused, indicate number of times.
  1. ☐ Hollow Fiber _____   3. ☐ Coil _____
  2. ☐ Parallel Plate _____   4. ☐ Other _____

	CAPD	Other
	1	2
j. Number of back-up sessions furnished to home patients		

HOME PROGRAM

k. Is Home Program Dialysis reimbursed under Target Rate Election?   ☐ Yes   ☐ No

l. Type of dialyzers used. If dialyzers are reused, indicate number of times.
  1. ☐ Hollow Fiber _____   3. ☐ Coil _____
  2. ☐ Parallel Plate _____   4. ☐ Other _____

2 Renal Dialysis Department—Number of Employees (Full Time Equivalents)

	Enter the number of hours in your normal work week _____	STAFF	CONTRACT	OTHER
		1	2	3
a. Physicians				
b. Registered Nurses				
c. Licensed Practical Nurses				
d. Nurses Aides				
e. Technicians				
f. Social Workers				
g. Dieticians				
h. Administrative				
i. Management				
j. Other (Specify)				

Exhibit 6

Exhibit 6 continued

WORKSHEET A Continued

PROVIDER NO

RECLASSIFICATION AND ADJUSTMENT OF TRIAL BALANCE OF EXPENSES

39	Medical Supplies Charged to Patients					
40	Drugs Charged to Patients					
41	Renal Dialysis					
42	Kidney Acquisition					
43						
44						
45	INPATIENT ROUTINE SERVICE COST CENTERS					
46	Adults & Pediatrics (General Routine Care)					
47	Intensive Care Unit					
48	Coronary Care Unit					
49						
50						
51	Nursery					
52	Skilled Nursing Facility—Certified					
53	Skilled Nursing Facility—Noncertified					
54	OUTPATIENT SERVICE COST CENTERS					
55	Clinic					
56	Emergency					
57						
58	OTHER REIMBURSABLE COST CENTERS					
59	Home Program Dialysis—Other					
60	Administrative & General—HHA					
61	Skilled Nursing Care—HHA					
62	Medical Social Services—HHA					
63	Home Health Aide—HHA					
64	Medical Appliances—HHA/DME-Rented					
65	Durable Medical Equipment Sold					
66	Home Delivered Meals—HHA					
67	Other Home Health Services—HHA					
68	Home Program Dialysis Equipment— 100% Medicare					
69	Ambulance Services					
70	Intern-Resident Service (not in approved teaching program)					
71	Malpractice Premiums and Paid Losses	-0-				
72	Interest Expense	-0-				
73	Utilization Review—SNF	-0-				
74	PSRO—Federal or Combined	-0-				
75	PSRO—Non Federal	-0-				
76						
77	SUBTOTAL (Sum of lines 2-76)	$	$	$	$	$
78	NONREIMBURSABLE COST CENTERS					
79	Gift, Flower, Coffee Shops & Canteen					
80	Research					
81	Physicians' Private Offices					
82	Nonpaid Workers					
83			-0-			
84	TOTAL (Sum of lines 77-83)	$	$	$	$	$

(1) Transfer the amounts in column 7 to Worksheet B, column 1

FORM HCFA-2552-81 (11-81)

6 continued

Exhibit 7

FORM APPROVED
OMB NO. 0938-0050

WORKSHEET A-1

RECLASSIFICATIONS AFFECTING ADMINISTRATIVE AND GENERAL EXPENSES

PROVIDER NO.

PERIOD: FROM / TO

ITEM	DEPRECIATION BUILDINGS & FIXTURES 1	DEPRECIATION MOVABLE EQUIPMENT 2	EMPLOYEE HEALTH & WELFARE 3	ADMINISTRATIVE & GENERAL 4	INTEREST EXPENSE 5	UTILIZATION REVIEW—SNF 6
1 Employee Health & Welfare benefits included in Administrative and General						
2 Personnel Department			$			
3 Employee Health Service						
4 Hospitalization Insurance						
5 Workmen's Compensation						
6 Employee Group Insurance						
7 Social Security Taxes						
8 Unemployment Taxes						
9 Annuity Premiums, Past Service Benefits, Pensions						
10						
11						
12						
13 Total employee benefit costs included in Administrative & General (Sum of lines 2–12)			$	$ ( )		
14 Insurance	$	$		( )	$( )	
15 Interest				( )	( )	
16 Rent				( )	( )	
17 Taxes (Real Property Taxes) (Personal Property Taxes)						
18 Utilization Review—SNF					$( )	$( )
19 TOTAL RECLASSIFICATIONS (Sum of lines 13–18) (Total of columns 1–6, line 19, should equal 0)	$	$	$	$ ( )	$ ( )	$ ( )
	TRANSFER TO WORKSHEET A, COL. 4, LINE 2	TRANSFER TO WORKSHEET A, COL. 4, LINE 3	TRANSFER TO WORKSHEET A, COL. 4, LINE 4	TRANSFER TO WORKSHEET A, COL. 4, LINE 5	TRANSFER TO WORKSHEET A, COL. 4, LINE 72	TRANSFER TO WORKSHEET A, COL. 4, LINE 73

7

FORM HCFA-2553-81 (11-81)

Exhibit 8

FORM APPROVED
OMB NO 0938-0050

RECLASSIFICATIONS OF DIETARY EXPENSE

PROVIDER NO _____

PERIOD
FROM _____
TO _____

WORKSHEET A-2

PART I — RECLASSIFICATION OF EXPENSES

	DESCRIPTION	TOTAL EXPENSES (FROM WKST A, COL 3, LINE AS INDICATED) 1	ANALYSIS OF DIETARY EXPENSES 2	TOTAL (SUM OF COLS. 1 & 2) 3	ALLOCATION OF TOTAL UNIDENTIFIED DIETARY EXPENSES	
					RATIO 4	AMOUNT 5
1	Dietary (From Worksheet A, col 3, line 10)		$			COL. 4, LINE 2 × COL. 2, LINE 7
2	Identified Expenses (1) Dietary (2)	(LINE 11)	$	$	COL. 3, LINE 2 ÷ COL. 3, LINE 6	COL. 4, LINE 3 × COL. 2, LINE 7
3	Cafeteria	$			COL. 3, LINE 3 ÷ COL. 3, LINE 6	COL. 4, LINE 4 × COL. 2, LINE 7
4					COL. 3, LINE 4 ÷ COL. 3, LINE 6	COL. 4, LINE 5 × COL. 2, LINE 7
5					COL. 3, LINE 5 ÷ COL. 3, LINE 6	
6	TOTAL (Sum of lines 2-5)	$	$	$	1.00000000	$
7	Unidentified Dietary Expenses (line 1 minus line 6)		$			

PART II — TRANSFER OF RECLASSIFIED EXPENSES

	ITEM	AMOUNT
1	Cafeteria (line 3, sum of columns 2 and 5) (Add on Worksheet A, column 4, line 11)	$
2	(line 4, sum of columns 2 and 5) (Add on Worksheet A, column 4, line as appropriate)	
3	(line 5, sum of columns 2 and 5) (Add on Worksheet A, column 4, line as appropriate)	
4	TOTAL (Sum of lines 1–3) (Deduct on Worksheet A, column 4, line 10)	$

(1) These amounts must be specifically identifiable in the accounting records or by analysis.

(2) Include in the dietary cost center all activities served directly from the dietary department; e.g., hospital inpatients, skilled nursing facility inpatients. If no cafeteria exists and employees and student nurses are served meals directly from the dietary department, costs for these items should be included in the dietary cost center and allocated to the proper departments on Worksheet B.

FORM HCFA-2552-81 (11-81)

8

Exhibit 9

FORM APPROVED
OMB NO 0938-0050

RECLASSIFICATION OF CENTRAL SERVICES & SUPPLY	PROVIDER NO	PERIOD: FROM _____ TO _____	WORKSHEET A-3

	ITEM	AMOUNT
1	Intern-Resident Service—(in approved teaching program) (Add on Worksheet A, column 4, line 19)	$
2	Intern-Resident Service—(not in approved teaching program) (Add on Worksheet A, column 4, line 70)	
3	Intravenous Therapy (Add on Worksheet A, column 4, line 32)	
4	Oxygen (Inhalation) Therapy (Add on Worksheet A, column 4, line 33)	
5		
6		
7	TOTAL (Sum of lines 1–6) (Deduct on Worksheet A, col. 4, line 14)	$

RECLASSIFICATION OF LABORATORY EXPENSE	PROVIDER NO	PERIOD: FROM _____ TO _____	WORKSHEET A-4

	ITEM	AMOUNT
1	Whole Blood and Packed Red Blood Cells (Add on Worksheet A, column 4, line 30)	$
2	Blood Storing, Processing & Transfusion (Add on Worksheet A, column 4, line 31)	
3	Electrocardiology (Add on Worksheet A, column 4, line 37)	
4	Electroencephalography (Add on Worksheet A, column 4, line 38)	
5		
6		
7	TOTAL (Sum of lines 1–6) (Deduct on Worksheet A, col. 4, line 29)	$

RECLASSIFICATION OF RADIOLOGY DIAGNOSTIC	PROVIDER NO	PERIOD: FROM _____ TO _____	WORKSHEET A-5

	ITEM	AMOUNT
1	Radiology—Therapeutic (Add on Worksheet A, column 4, line 27)	$
2	Radioisotope (Add on Worksheet A, column 4, line 28)	
3	Electrocardiology (Add on Worksheet A, column 4, line 37)	
4	Electroencephalography (Add on Worksheet A, column 4, line 38)	
5		
6		
7	TOTAL (Sum of lines 1–6) (Deduct on Worksheet A, col. 4, line 26)	$

Exhibit 10

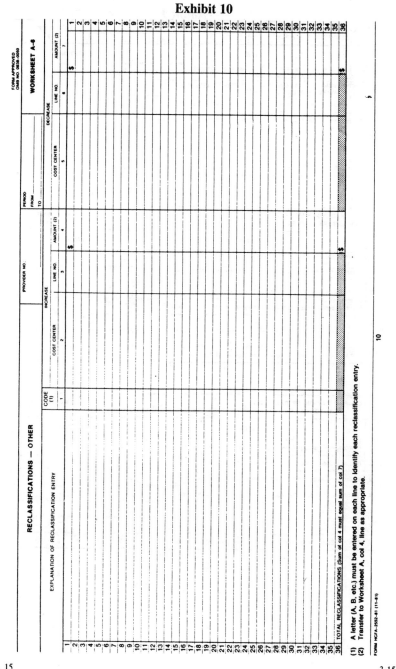

Exhibit 11

FORM APPROVED
OMB NO. 0938-0050

WORKSHEET A-7

PROVIDER NO. _____

PERIOD
FROM _____
TO _____

LIMITATION ON FEDERAL PARTICIPATION FOR CAPITAL EXPENDITURES QUESTIONNAIRE

1 Analysis of changes during cost reporting period in capital asset balances of components certified to participate in health care programs.

DESCRIPTION	BEGINNING BALANCE 1	ACQUISITIONS PURCHASE 2	ACQUISITIONS DONATION 3	TOTAL 4	DISPOSALS AND RETIREMENTS 5	ENDING BALANCE 6
Land	$	$	$	$	$( )	$
Land Improvements					( )	
Buildings & Fixtures					( )	
Building Improvements					( )	
Equipment						
Fixed					( )	
Movable					( )	
TOTAL	$	$	$	$	$( )	$

2 Were there any obligations and/or expenditures incurred for capital expenditures (as defined in Provider Reimbursement Manual Part I, chapter 24) by or on behalf of the provider during the period to which this cost report applies and subsequent to (1) December 31, 1972, or (2) the effective date of the agreement between the State and the Secretary, whichever is later.

☐ YES   ☐ NO   *If "No", DO NOT COMPLETE THE REMAINDER OF THIS WORKSHEET.*

3 Enter the following data relative to each capital expenditure (as defined in Provider Reimbursement Manual Part I, chapter 24) made by or on behalf of the provider during the period to which this cost report applies and subsequent to (1) December 31, 1972, or (2) the effective date of the agreement between the State and the Secretary, whichever is later.

DESCRIPTION	HOW ACQUIRED: ENTER LETTER SYMBOL (1) 1	DATE OBLIGATION INCURRED 2	COST 3	EXPENSES INCLUDED ON WKST A, COL. 5, RELATED TO CAPITAL EXPENDITURES DEPRECIATION 4	INTEREST 5	RENT 6	OTHER EXPENSE 7	OTHER AMOUNT 8	TOTAL (SUM OF COLS 4, 5, 6, 8) 9
a.			$	$	$	$	$	$	$
b.			$	$	$	$	$	$	$
c.			$	$	$	$	$	$	$
d.									

4 Enter the following data with regard to the provider's written notice of intention to make each capital expenditure described in item 3 above. The capital expenditures should be listed in the same chronological order as those listed in item 3.

DESCRIPTION	DATE WRITTEN NOTICE SUBMITTED 1	DATE APPROVED 2	DATE OF NOTICE OF DISAPPROVAL REC'D 3	APPEAL OF DENIAL DATE 4	STATUS OF APPEAL 5
a.					
b.					
c.					
d.					

(1) Use the following symbols to indicate how the asset was acquired.
A—Purchase on the open market
B—Donation or transfer
C—Lease or comparable arrangement

FORM HCFA-2552-81 (11-81)

11

Exhibit 12

FORM APPROVED
OMB NO. 0938–0050

ADJUSTMENTS TO EXPENSES	PROVIDER NO.:	PERIOD: FROM _____ TO _____	WORKSHEET A–8

DESCRIPTION (1)	BASIS FOR ADJUST-MENT (2)	AMOUNT	EXPENSE CLASSIFICATION ON WORKSHEET A FROM WHICH THE AMOUNT IS TO BE DEDUCTED OR TO WHICH THE AMOUNT IS TO BE ADDED	
			COST CENTER	LINE NO
	1	2	3	4
1. Investment income on commingled restricted and unrestricted funds (chapter 2)		$		
2. Trade, quantity, and time discounts on purchases (chapter 8)				
3. Rebates and refunds of expenses (chapter 8)				
4. Rental of provider space by suppliers (chapter 8)				
5. Telephone service (pay stations excluded) (chapter 21)				
6. Television and radio service (chapter 21)				
7. Parking lot (chapter 21)				
8. Remuneration applicable to provider-based radiologists for professional services (chapter 21)				
9. Remuneration applicable to provider-based pathologists for professional services (chapter 21)				
10. Remuneration applicable to provider-based anesthesiologists for professional services (chapter 21)				
11. Remuneration applicable to provider-based cardiologists for professional services (chapter 21)				
12. Remuneration applicable to provider-based neurologists for professional services (chapter 21)				
13.				
14.				
15.				
16.				
17. Home office costs (chapter 21)				
18. Sale of scrap, waste, etc. (chapter 23)				
19. Nonallowable costs related to certain capital expenditures (chapter 24)				
20. Adjustment resulting from transactions with related organizations (chapter 10)	Fr Wkst A–8–1			
21. Laundry and linen service				
22. Cafeteria—employees, guests, etc.				
23. Rental of living quarters to employees and others				
24. Sale of medical and surgical supplies to other than patients				
25. Sale of drugs to other than patients				
26. Sale of medical records and abstracts				
27. Nursing school (tuition, fees, textbooks, uniforms, etc.)				
28. Vending machines				
29. Income from imposition of interest, finance or penalty charges (chapter 21)				
30.				
31.				
32. SUBTOTAL (Sum of lines 1–31) (Carry forward to page 13, Worksheet A-8, line 33)		$		

(1) Description—all line references in this column pertain to the Provider Reimbursement Manual, Part I.

(2) Basis for adjustment (SEE INSTRUCTIONS).
   A. Costs—if cost, including applicable overhead, can be determined.
   B. Amount Received—if cost cannot be determined.

FORM HCFA-2552-81 (11–81)   12

Exhibit 12 continued

FORM APPROVED
OMB NO. 0938-0050

ADJUSTMENTS TO EXPENSES			PROVIDER NO:		PERIOD: FROM _____ TO _____		WORKSHEET A-8
	DESCRIPTION (1)	BASIS FOR ADJUST-MENT (2)	AMOUNT		EXPENSE CLASSIFICATION ON WORKSHEET A FROM WHICH THE AMOUNT IS TO BE DEDUCTED OR TO WHICH THE AMOUNT IS TO BE ADDED		
					COST CENTER		LINE NO
		1	2		3		4
33.	SUBTOTAL (Brought forward from page 12, Worksheet A-8, line 32)		$				
34.	Adjustment For Physical Therapy costs in excess of limitation (Chapter 14)	From Supple-mental Work-sheet A-8-3	( )				
35.	Malpractice Premiums and/or Self-Ins. Fund Contributions (Chapter 21)						
36.	Allowable Paid Title XVIII Malpractice Losses (Chapter 21)						
37.	Allowable Related Direct Expenses to Paid Title XVIII Malpractice Losses (Chapter 21)						
38.	Allowable Paid Title XIX Malpractice Losses (Chapter 21)						
39.	Allowable Related Direct Expenses to Paid Title XIX Malpractice Losses (Chapter 21)						
40.	Allowable Paid Title V Malpractice Losses (Chapter 21)						
41.	Allowable Related Direct Expenses to Paid Title V Malpractice Losses (Chapter 21)						
42.	Allowable Paid Malpractice Losses & Related Direct Exp. Appl. to the Home Health Ag'cy.						
43.	Nonallowable Malpractice Premiums, Paid Losses and Related Expenses (Chapter 21)						
44.							
45.	PSRO Costs (Federal or Combined) (HCFA Pub. 15-I, 1975 Amendments)						
46.	PSRO Costs (Non-Federal Only) (HCFA Pub. 15-I, 1975 Amendments)						
47.							
48.							
49.							
50.							
51.							
52.							
53.							
54.							
55.							
56.							
57.							
58.	SUBTOTAL (Sum of lines 33-57)		$				
59.	Grants, gifts, and income designated by donor for specific expenses (chapter 6)						
60.	Utilization review—physicians' compensation (chapter 21)						
61.	Depreciation—buildings and fixtures						
62.	Depreciation—movable equipment						
63.							
64.	TOTAL (line 58 plus or minus the sum of lines 59-63) (Transfer to Worksheet A, col. 6, line 84)		$				

(1) Description—all line references in this column pertain to HCFA Pub. 15-I.
(2) Basis for adjustment (SEE INSTRUCTIONS).
    A. Costs—if cost, including applicable overhead, can be determined.
    B. Amount Received—if cost cannot be determined.

Exhibit 13

FORM APPROVED
OMB NO. 0938—0050

| STATEMENT OF COSTS OF SERVICES FROM RELATED ORGANIZATIONS | PROVIDER NO | PERIOD FROM ___ TO ___ | WORKSHEET A–8–1 |

A. Are there any costs included on Worksheet A which resulted from transactions with related organizations as defined in HCFA Pub. 15–1, chapter 10?

☐ Yes   ☐ No   (If "Yes," complete Parts B and C)

B. Costs incurred and adjustment required as result of transactions with related organizations:

	LOCATION AND AMOUNT INCLUDED ON WORKSHEET A. COLUMN 5			AMOUNT ALLOWABLE IN COST	NET ADJUSTMENTS (COL. 4 MINUS COL. 5)
LINE NO.	COST CENTER	EXPENSE ITEMS	AMOUNT		
1	2	3	4	5	6
1.			$	$	$
2.					
3.					
4.					
5.	TOTALS (Sum of lines 1–4) (Transfer col 6, lines 1–4 to Wkst A, col. 6, lines as appropriate) (Transfer col. 6, line 5 to Wkst A–8, col. 2, line 20)		$	$	$

C. Interrelationship of provider to related organization(s):

The Secretary, by virtue of authority granted under Section 1814(b)(1) of the Social Security Act, requires the provider to furnish the information requested on Part C of this Worksheet.

The information will be used by the Health Care Financing Administration and its intermediaries in determining that the costs applicable to services, facilities and supplies furnished by organizations related to the provider by common ownership or control, represent reasonable costs as determined under Section 1861 of the Social Security Act. If the provider does not provide all or any part of the requested information, the cost report will be considered incomplete and not acceptable for purposes of claiming reimbursement under title XVIII.

			RELATED ORGANIZATION(S)		
SYMBOL (1)	NAME	PERCENT OWNERSHIP OF PROVIDER	NAME	PERCENT OF OWNERSHIP	TYPE OF BUSINESS
1	2	3	4	5	6
1.					
2.					
3.					
4.					
5.					

(1) Use the following symbols to indicate the interrelationship of the provider to related organizations

A Individual has financial interest (stockholder, partner, etc.) in both related organization and in provider
B Corporation, partnership, or other organization has financial interest in provider
C Provider has financial interest in corporation, partnership, or other organization
D Director, officer, administrator, or key person of provider or relative of such person has financial interest in related organization
E Individual is director, officer, administrator, or key person of provider and related organization
F Director, officer, administrator or key person of related organization or relative of such person has financial interest in provider
G Other (financial or non-financial) specify

| DEPRECIATION | PROVIDER NO | PERIOD FROM ___ TO ___ | WORKSHEET A–8–2 |

1 Depreciation reported in cost statement:

A. Straight-Line $ _____   C. Sum-of-the-Years' Digits _____

B. Declining Balance _____   D. Optional Allowance _____

E. Depreciation reported on Worksheet A, column 7 (Sum of A, B, C, and D) $ _____

		YES	NO
2	Is Depreciation Funded? (If Yes: Balance In Fund At End of Period $ _____)		
3	Were There Any Disposals of Capital Assets During Period?		
4	Was Accelerated Depreciation Claimed On Any Assets In The Current Or any Prior Cost Reporting Period?		
	If Yes: A. Was Accelerated Depreciation Claimed On Assets Acquired On Or After August 1, 1970? (See HCFA Pub. 15–1, Chapter 1)		
	B. Did Provider Cease To Participate In The Medicare Program At End Of Period To Which This Cost Report Applies? (See HCFA Pub. 15–1, Chapter 1)		
	C. Was There Substantial Decrease In Health Insurance Proportion Of Allowable Costs From Prior Cost Reporting Periods? (See HCFA Pub. 15–1, Chapter 1)		

FORM HCFA-2552-81 (11-81)   14

Medicare Regulations Regarding the Hospital Cost Allocation Process

The following Medicare instructions apply, at this writing, to the hospital cost allocation process, as discussed in Chapter 5. Relevant worksheets, identified by exhibit number from the list of worksheets in Appendix F, follow the instructions. Cost allocation techniques are applied on Medicare Worksheet B and Worksheet B-1. These are commonly called the Medicare Stepdown schedules.

Lines 1A, 1B, 1C and 1D--Indicate on the appropriate line, the
amount of depreciation claimed under each method of depreciation
used by the provider during the cost reporting period.

Line 1E--The total depreciation shown on line 1E will not equal
the amount shown on Worksheet E, column 7, lines 2 and 3, for
depreciation, but represents the amount of depreciation included
in costs on Worksheet A, column 7.

328.   WORKSHEET B - COST ALLOCATION - GENERAL SERVICES COSTS AND
       WORKSHEET B-1 - COST ALLOCATION - STATISTICAL BASIS
Worksheet B provides for the allocation of the expenses of each
general service cost center to those cost centers which receive
the services. The cost centers serviced by the general service
cost centers include all cost centers within the provider organization; that is, other general service cost centers, ancillary
service cost centers, inpatient routine service cost centers,
outpatient service cost centers, other reimbursable cost centers
and nonreimbursable cost centers. The total direct expenses are
obtained from Worksheet A, column 7.

Worksheet B-1 provides for the proration of the statistical data
needed to equitably allocate the expenses of the general service
cost centers on Worksheet B.

To facilitate the allocation process, the general format of
Worksheets B and B-1 are identical. Each general service cost
center has the same line number as its respective column number
across the top. Also, the column and line numbers for each
general service cost center are identical on the two worksheets.
In addition, the line numbers for each ancillary, routine, other
reimbursable and nonreimbursable cost centers are identical on
the two worksheets.

The statistical bases shown at the top of each column on
Worksheet B-1 are the recommended bases of allocation of the cost
centers indicated.

Most cost centers are allocated on different statistical bases.
However, for those cost centers where the basis is the same
(e.g., square feet), the total statistical base over which the
costs are to be allocated will differ because of the prior
elimination of cost centers that have been closed.

When closing the general service cost centers, first close
those cost centers that render the most services to and receive
the least services from other cost centers. The cost centers
are listed in this sequence from left to right on the worksheets.
However, the circumstances of a provider may be such that a more
accurate result is obtained by allocating to certain cost centers
in a sequence different from that followed on these worksheets.

NOTE: A provider wishing to change its allocation basis for a
        particular cost center or the order in which the cost
        centers are allocated must make a written request to its
        intermediary for approval of the change and submit reason-
        able justification for such change prior to the beginning
        of the cost reporting period for which the change is to
        apply. The effective date of the change will be the
        beginning of the cost reporting period for which the
        request has been made. (See PRM, Part I, chapter 23.)

If the amount of any cost center on Worksheet A, column 7, has a
credit balance, this amount must be shown as a credit balance on
Worksheet B, column 1. The costs from the applicable overhead
cost centers will be allocated in the normal manner to such cost
center showing a credit balance. After receiving costs from the
applicable overhead cost centers, if a general service cost center
has a credit balance at the point it is to be allocated, such
general service cost center must not be allocated. Rather, the
credit balance is entered in parenthesis on an unspecified
nonreimbursable cost center line (i.e., line 73) as well as the
first line of the column and line 74. This will enable
column 21, line 74, to crossfoot to columns 1 and 4a, line 74.
After receiving costs from the applicable overhead cost centers,
if a revenue-producing cost center has a credit balance on
Worksheet B, column 21, such credit balance will not be carried
forward to Worksheet C.

If the specific operating costs to which a grant, gift or
endowment income, designated by the donor for specific expenses,
is to be applied constitute a general service cost center and
such cost center still has a credit balance at the point it is
to be allocated in the cost finding process, such credit balance
should not be allocated. Rather, it should be entered in parenthesis on an unspecified nonreimbursable cost center line (i.e.,
line 73) as well as the first line of the column and line 74.
This will enable column 21, line 74, to crossfoot to columns 1
and 4a, line 74. Such credit balance should be carried forward
and applied in the succeeding cost reporting period as an
adjustment to expenses on Worksheet A-8 unless the donor stipulated that the grant is for the current cost reporting period
only, thereby the excess is free from restriction and not
carried forward to the succeeding year as an adjustment to
expenses.

If the specific operating costs to which a grant, gift or
endowment income, designated by donor for specific expenses, is
to be applied constitute a revenue-producing cost center and
such cost center has a credit balance on Worksheet B, column 21,
after receiving overhead allocations through the cost finding
process, such credit balance will not be carried forward to
Worksheet C. Such credit balance should be carried forward and

applied in the succeeding cost reporting period as an adjustment
to expenses on Worksheet A-8 unless the donor stipulated that the
amount of the grant is for the current cost reporting period only,
thereby the excess is free from restriction and not carried
forward to the succeeding year as an adjustment to expenses.

On Worksheet B-1, enter on the first line in the column of the
cost center being allocated, the total statistical base over
which the expenses are to be allocated (e.g., column 2 -
Depreciation - Buildings and Fixtures, enter on line 2 the total
square feet of the buildings and fixtures on which depreciation
was taken).

Such statistical base should not include any statistics related
to services furnished under arrangements except where:

        1. both Medicare and non-Medicare costs of arranged-for
services are recorded in the provider's records or

        2. the intermediary determines that the provider is
able to "gross up" the costs and charges for services to
non-Medicare patients so that both costs and charges are recorded
as if the provider had furnished such services directly to all
patients - Medicare and non-Medicare. (See PRM, Part I, chapter 23.)

For all cost centers (below the first line) to which the
depreciation is being allocated, enter that portion of the total
statistical base applicable to each. The total sum of the
statistical base applied to each cost center receiving the
services rendered must equal the total base entered on the first
line.

Enter on line 74, the total expenses of the cost center to be
allocated. This amount is obtained from Worksheet B, from the
same column and line number used to enter the total statistical
base on Worksheet B-1 (in the case of Buildings and Fixtures
depreciation, this amount is on Worksheet B, column 2, line 2).

Divide the amount entered on line 74 by the total statistical
base entered in the same column on the first line. Enter the
resulting Unit Cost Multiplier on line 75. The Unit Cost
Multiplier must show at least eight decimal places.

Multiply the Unit Cost Multiplier by that portion of the total
statistical base applicable to each cost center receiving the
services rendered. Enter the result of each computation on
Worksheet B in the corresponding column and line.

After the Unit Cost Multiplier has been applied to all the cost
centers receiving the services rendered, the total expenses
(line 74) of all of the cost centers receiving the allocation
on Worksheet B must equal the amount entered on the first line.

The preceding procedures must be performed for each general service cost center. Each cost center must be completed on both Worksheets B and B-1 before proceeding to the next cost center.

After all the costs of the general service cost centers have been allocated on Worksheet B, enter in column 21, the sum of expenses on lines 22 through 73, columns 4a through 20. The total expenses entered in column 21, line 74, should equal the total expenses entered in column 1, line 74.

Transfer the totals in column 21, lines 22 through 41 and lines 43 and 44 (ancillary service cost centers), lines 55 through 57 (outpatient service cost centers), and lines 59 through 63 (other reimbursable cost centers) to Worksheet C, column 1, lines 2a through 32a (above the dotted rules).

NOTE: If the provider furnishes outpatient renal dialysis services and uses either an inpatient routine bed, or a bed or other accommodation in the outpatient area (other than in the renal dialysis department) to furnish such services, the amount in column 21, line 41, will not be transferred to Worksheet C, column 1, line 21a. Instead, this amount should be transferred to Supplemental Worksheet D-7, Part III, line 2.

Transfer the total in column 21, line 42, to Supplemental Worksheet D-6, Part I, line 5.

Transfer the totals in column 21, lines 46 through 52, to Worksheet D-1, column and line, as follows:

From Worksheet B, column 21	To Worksheet D-1
Line 46 (hospital)	Column 1, line 11
Line 47 (intensive care unit)	Column 1, line 40
Line 48 (coronary care unit)	Column 1, line 41
Line 49 (subprovider) or	Column 2 or 3, line 11
Line 49 (special care unit)	Column 1, line 42
Line 50 (subprovider) or	Column 2 or 3, line 11
Line 50 (special care unit)	Column 1, line 43
Line 51 (nursery)	Column 1, 2 or 3, line 54
Line 52 (skilled nursing facility - certified)	Column 4, line 11

Transfer the total expenses in column 21, line 64 (Home Program Dialysis Equipment - 100% Medicare) to Worksheet E, Part III, line 13.

Transfer the total expenses in column 21, line 65 (Ambulance
Services) to Supplemental Worksheet D-5, line 1.

Transfer the total expenses in column 21, line 66 (Intern-
Resident Services Not In Approved Teaching Program) to
Worksheet D-2, Part I, column 2, line 1.

The nonreimbursable cost center totals, lines 69 through 73, are
not transferred.

NOTE: Whenever an adjustment is required to expenses after
        cost allocation, the provider must submit a supporting
        worksheet showing the computation of the adjustment,
        the amount applicable to each cost center, and the cost
        center balances which are to be carried forward from
        Worksheet B for cost apportionment to the health care
        programs.

Some examples of adjustments which may be required to expenses
after cost allocation are: (1) the allocation of standby costs
between the certified portion and the noncertified portion of a
distinct-part provider and (2) costs attributable to unoccupied
beds of a provider with a restrictive admission policy. (See
PRM, Part I, chapter 23.)

COLUMN DESCRIPTIONS

Column 2 - Depreciation - Buildings and Fixtures--Depreciation
on buildings and fixtures and expenses pertaining to buildings
and fixtures such as insurance, interest, rent and real estate
taxes are combined in this cost center to facilitate cost
allocation.

Column 3 - Depreciation - Movable Equipment--Providers that do
not directly assign the depreciation on movable equipment and
expenses pertaining to movable equipment such as insurance,
interest and rent as part of their normal accounting systems
must accumulate the expenses in this cost center.

Column 5 - Administrative and General--The administrative and
general expenses are allocated on the basis of accumulated costs.
Therefore, the amount to be entered on Worksheet B-1, column 5,
line 5, is the sum of (1) the difference between the amounts
entered on line 74 and line 5 on Worksheet B, column 4a, plus
(2) the adjustment for grants, gifts and income designated by
donor for specific expenses entered on Worksheet A-8, line 59.

The amounts to be entered on Worksheet B-1, column 5, lines 6
through 73, are obtained from Worksheet B, column 4a, lines 6
through 73, after these have been increased by the amounts
appearing on Worksheet A-8, line 59. If adjustments to expenses
were made on Worksheet A-8, line 59, the provider must attach a

supporting worksheet showing the computation of the amounts entered
on Worksheet B-1, column 5, lines 6 through 73. That cost,
which was reduced by the grant, must be fully reflected in the
appropriate cost center(s) in this column to receive a fair
share of administrative and general expense.

A negative cost center balance in the statistics for allocating
administrative and general expenses causes an improper distribution of this overhead cost center. Negative balances must be
excluded from the allocation statistics when administrative and
general expenses are allocated on the basis of accumulated cost.

On the other hand, in arriving at the amounts entered in the
subtotal column of Worksheet B before allocation of administrative
and general expenses (column 4a) some cost centers may have
negative balances caused by offsets of grants, gifts or endowment
income. In this situation, the full amount of such offsets to
these cost centers is restored to the balances before they are
entered on Worksheet B-1, column 5, as allocation statistics for
the administrative and general cost center. After the restoration
of offsets due to grants, gifts and endowment income, and there
is still a negative balance, exclude the negative balance from
the allocation statistics when the administrative and general
expenses are allocated on the basis of accumulated cost.

330. WORKSHEET C - DEPARTMENTAL COST DISTRIBUTION
On this worksheet the lines in column 1 and columns 3 through 10
are divided by a dotted rule into two parts: Part a and Part b.
In each instance, cost data is entered in Part b.

THE PROVIDER SHOULD SUBMIT ALL DATA REQUESTED IN COLUMNS 1 THROUGH
10, LINES 1 THROUGH 33, AS APPROPRIATE.

Column 1--Enter on Part a of each line, the total cost of each cost
center as computed on Worksheet B, column 21, lines 22 through
41, 43 and 44, 55 through 57 and 59 through 63. Exceptions:
(1) When adjustments to expenses are required after cost allocation
(e.g., adjustments needed for allocation of standby costs or
adjustments for costs applicable to unoccupied beds of a provider
with a restrictive admission policy), the adjusted cost center
expenses to be entered on Worksheet C must be obtained from the
supporting worksheet submitted by the provider. See the instructions for completing Worksheet B; (2) Providers that furnish
outpatient renal dialysis services and use either an inpatient
routine bed, or a bed or other accommodation in the outpatient area
(other than in the renal dialysis department) to furnish this
service must adjust the renal dialysis cost computed on
Worksheet B, column 21, line 41. In this instance, adjusted renal
dialysis cost to be entered on line 21a is obtained from
Supplemental Worksheet D-7, Part III, line 3; (3) Any cost center
with a credit balance is not brought forward from Worksheet B,

Exhibit 14

FORM APPROVED
OMB NO 0938-0050

WORKSHEET B

COST ALLOCATION—GENERAL SERVICE COSTS

PROVIDER NO _____   PERIOD FROM _____ TO _____

COST CENTER (OMIT CENTS)	NET EXPENSES FOR COST ALLOCATION (FROM WKST A, COLUMN 7) 1	DEPRECIATION BUILDINGS & FIXTURES 2	DEPRECIATION MOVABLE EQUIPMENT 3	EMPLOYEE HEALTH & WELFARE 4	SUBTOTAL (COLS 1-4) 4a	ADMINISTRATIVE & GENERAL 5	MAINTENANCE & REPAIRS 6	OPERATION OF PLANT 7	
GENERAL SERVICE COST CENTERS									1
Depreciation—Buildings & Fixtures									2
Depreciation—Movable Equipment									3
Employee Health & Welfare									4
Administrative & General									5
Maintenance & Repairs									6
Operation of Plant									7
Laundry & Linen Service									8
Housekeeping									9
Dietary									10
Cafeteria									11
Maintenance of Personnel									12
Nursing Administration									13
Central Services & Supply									14
Pharmacy									15
Medical Records & Library									16
Social Service									17
Nursing School									18
Intern-Resident Service (in approved teaching program)									19
									20
ANCILLARY SERVICE COST CENTERS									21
Operating Room									22
Recovery Room									23
Delivery Room & Labor Room									24
Anesthesiology									25
Radiology-Diagnostic									26
Radiology—Therapeutic									27
Radioisotope									28
Laboratory									29
Whole Blood and Packed Red Blood Cells									30
Blood Storing, Processing and Transfusion									31
Intravenous Therapy									32
Oxygen (Inhalation) Therapy									33
Physical Therapy									34
Occupational Therapy									35
Speech Pathology									36

FORM HCFA-2552-81 (11-81)

15

Exhibit 14 continued

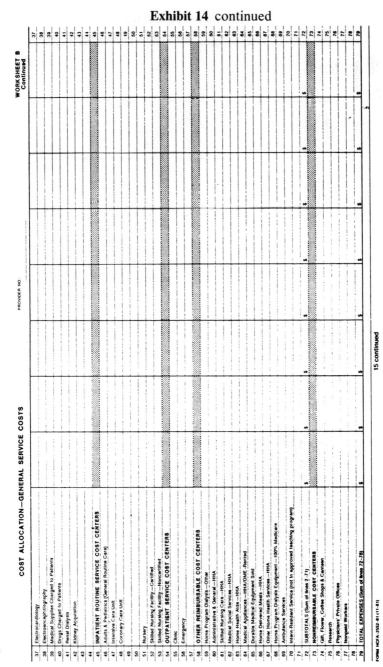

WORKSHEET B
Continued

PROVIDER NO.

COST ALLOCATION—GENERAL SERVICE COSTS

37	Electrocardiology	37
38	Electroencephalography	38
39	Medical Supplies Charged to Patients	39
40	Drugs Charged to Patients	40
41	Renal Dialysis	41
42	Kidney Acquisition	42
43		43
44		44
45	INPATIENT ROUTINE SERVICE COST CENTERS	45
46	Adults & Pediatrics (General Routine Care)	46
47	Intensive Care Unit	47
48	Coronary Care Unit	48
49		49
50		50
51	Nursery	51
52	Skilled Nursing Facility—Certified	52
53	Skilled Nursing Facility—Noncertified	53
54	OUTPATIENT SERVICE COST CENTERS	54
55	Clinic	55
56	Emergency	56
57		57
58	OTHER REIMBURSABLE COST CENTERS	58
59	Home Program Dialysis—Other	59
60	Administrative & General—HHA	60
61	Skilled Nursing Care—HHA	61
62	Medical Social Services—HHA	62
63	Home Health Aide—HHA	63
64	Medical Appliances—HHA/DME-Rented	64
65	Durable Medical Equipment Sold	65
66	Home Delivered Meals—HHA	66
67	Other Home Health Services—HHA	67
68	Home Program Dialysis Equipment—100% Medicare	68
69	Ambulance Services	69
70	Intern-Resident Service (not in approved teaching program)	70
71		71
72	SUBTOTALS (Sum of lines 2 -71)	72
73	NONREIMBURSABLE COST CENTERS	73
74	Gift, Flower, Coffee Shops & Canteen	74
75	Research	75
76	Physicians' Private Offices	76
77	Nonpaid Workers	77
78		78
79	TOTAL EXPENSES (Sum of lines 72-78)	79

FORM HCFA-2552-81(11-81)

15 continued

Exhibit 14 continued

COST ALLOCATION—GENERAL SERVICE COSTS

WORKSHEET B

FORM APPROVED
OMB NO. 0938-0050

PROVIDER NO

PERIOD: FROM ___ TO ___

COST CENTER (COST CENTS)	LAUNDRY & LINEN SERVICE	HOUSEKEEPING	DIETARY	CAFETERIA	MAINTENANCE OF PERSONNEL	NURSING ADMINISTRATION	CENTRAL SERVICES & SUPPLY
	8	9	10	11	12	13	14

GENERAL SERVICE COST CENTERS
1
2 Depreciation—Buildings & Fixture
3 Depreciation—Movable Equipment
4 Employee Health & Welfare
5 Administrative & General
6 Maintenance & Repairs
7 Operation of Plant
8 Laundry & Linen Service
9 Housekeeping
10 Dietary
11 Cafeteria
12 Maintenance of Personnel
13 Nursing Administration
14 Central Services & Supply
15 Pharmacy
16 Medical Records & Library
17 Social Service
18 Nursing School
19 Intern-Resident Service (in approved teaching program)
20 ANCILLARY SERVICE COST CENTERS
21 Operating Room
22 Recovery Room
23 Delivery Room & Labor Room
24 Anesthesiology
25 Radiology—Diagnostic
26 Radiology—Therapeutic
27 Radioisotope
28 Laboratory
29 Whole Blood and Packed Red Blood Cells
30 Blood Storing, Processing and Transfusion
31 Intravenous Therapy
32 Oxygen (Inhalation) Therapy
33 Physical Therapy
34 Occupational Therapy
35 Speech Pathology

FORM HCFA-2552-81 (11-81)

16

Exhibit 14 continued

COST ALLOCATION—GENERAL SERVICE COSTS   PROVIDER NO.   WORKSHEET B Continued

37	Electrocardiology
38	Electroencephalography
39	Medical Supplies Charged to Patients
40	Drugs Charged to Patients
41	Renal Dialysis
42	Kidney Acquisition
43	
44	
45	**INPATIENT ROUTINE SERVICE COST CENTERS**
46	Adults & Pediatrics (General Routine Care)
47	Intensive Care Unit
48	Coronary Care Unit
49	
50	
51	Nursery
52	Skilled Nursing Facility—Certified
53	Skilled Nursing Facility—Noncertified
54	**OUTPATIENT SERVICE COST CENTERS**
55	Clinic
56	Emergency
57	
58	**OTHER REIMBURSABLE COST CENTERS**
59	Home Program Dialysis—Other
60	Administrative & General—HHA
61	Skilled Nursing Care—HHA
62	Medical Social Services—HHA
63	Home Health Aide—HHA
64	Medical Appliances—HHA/DME-Rented
65	Durable Medical Equipment Sold
66	Home Delivered Meals—HHA
67	Other Home Health Services—HHA
68	Home Program Dialysis Equipment—100% Medicare
69	Ambulance Services
70	Intern-Resident Service (not in approved teaching program)
71	
72	SUBTOTALS (Sum of lines 9-71)
73	**NONREIMBURSABLE COST CENTERS**
74	Gift, Flower, Coffee Shops & Canteen
75	Research
76	Physicians' Private Offices
77	Nonpaid Workers
78	
79	TOTAL EXPENSES (Sum of lines 72-78)

FORM HCFA-2552-81(11-83)

16 continued

Rev. 15

Exhibit 14 continued

Exhibit 14 continued

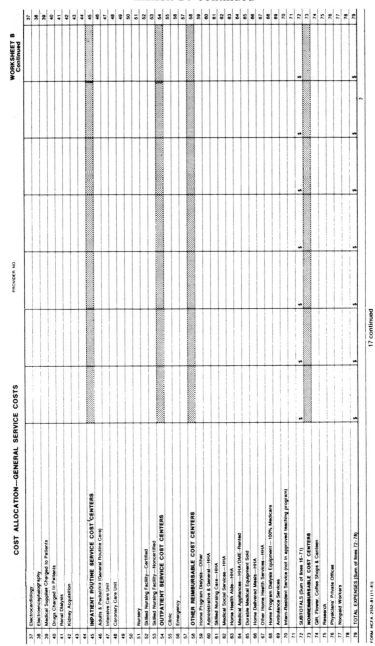

WORKSHEET B
Continued

PROVIDER NO.

COST ALLOCATION—GENERAL SERVICE COSTS

37	Electrocardiology
38	Electroencephalography
39	Medical Supplies Charged to Patients
40	Drugs Charged to Patients
41	Renal Dialysis
42	Kidney Acquisition
43	
44	
45	INPATIENT ROUTINE SERVICE COST CENTERS
46	Adults & Pediatrics (General Routine Care)
47	Intensive Care Unit
48	Coronary Care Unit
49	
50	
51	Nursery
52	Skilled Nursing Facility—Certified
53	Skilled Nursing Facility—Noncertified
54	OUTPATIENT SERVICE COST CENTERS
55	Clinic
56	Emergency
57	
58	OTHER REIMBURSABLE COST CENTERS
59	Home Program Dialysis—Other
60	Administrative & General—HHA
61	Skilled Nursing Care—HHA
62	Medical Social Services—HHA
63	Home Health Aide—HHA
64	Medical Appliances—HHA/DME-Rented
65	Durable Medical Equipment Sold
66	Home Delivered Meals—HHA
67	Other Home Health Services—HHA
68	Home Program Dialysis Equipment—100% Medicare
69	Ambulance Services
70	Intern-Resident Service (not in approved teaching program)
71	
72	SUBTOTALS (Sum of lines 16-71)
73	NONREIMBURSABLE COST CENTERS
74	Gift, Flower, Coffee Shops & Canteen
75	Research
76	Physicians' Private Offices
77	Nonpaid Workers
78	
79	TOTAL EXPENSES (Sum of lines 72-78)

FORM HCFA-2552-81 (11-81)

17 continued

Exhibit 15

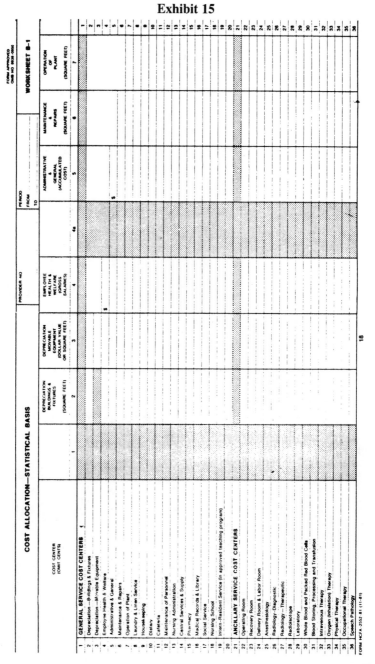

Exhibit 15 continued

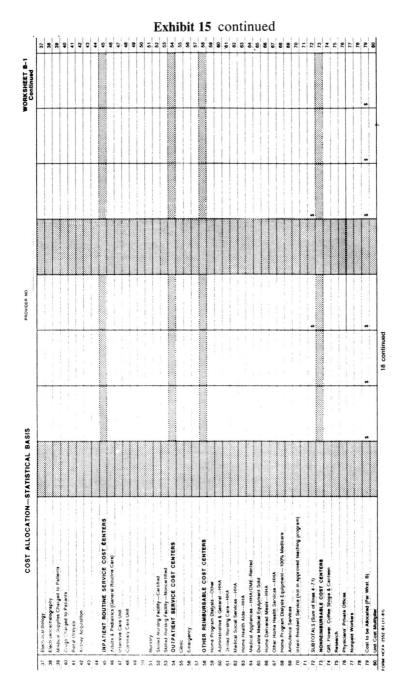

Exhibit 15 continued

FORM APPROVED
OMB NO. 0938-0050

WORKSHEET B-1

COST ALLOCATION—STATISTICAL BASIS

PROVIDER NO

PERIOD
FROM
TO

COST CENTER (OMIT CENTS)	LAUNDRY & LINEN SERVICE (POUNDS OF LAUNDRY)	HOUSEKEEPING (HOURS OF SERVICE)	DIETARY (MEALS SERVED)	CAFETERIA (MEALS SERVED)	MAINTENANCE OF PERSONNEL (NUMBER HOUSED)	NURSING ADMINISTRATION (DIRECT NURSING HOURS OF SERVICE)	CENTRAL SERVICES & SUPPLY (COSTED REQUISITIONS)	
	8	9	10	11	12	13	14	
GENERAL SERVICE COST CENTERS								1
2 Depreciation—Buildings & Fixtures								2
3 Depreciation—Movable Equipment								3
4 Employee Health & Welfare								4
5 Administrative & General								5
6 Maintenance & Repairs								6
7 Operation of Plant								7
8 Laundry & Linen Service								8
9 Housekeeping								9
10 Dietary								10
11 Cafeteria								11
12 Maintenance of Personnel								12
13 Nursing Administration								13
14 Central Services & Supply							$	14
15 Pharmacy								15
16 Medical Records & Library								16
17 Social Service								17
18 Nursing School								18
19 Intern-Resident Service (in approved teaching program)								19
20								20
21 **ANCILLARY SERVICE COST CENTERS**								21
22 Operating Room								22
23 Recovery Room								23
24 Delivery Room & Labor Room								24
25 Anesthesiology								25
26 Radiology—Diagnostic								26
27 Radiology—Therapeutic								27
28 Radioisotope								28
29 Laboratory								29
30 Whole Blood and Packed Red Blood Cells								30
31 Blood Storing, Processing and Transfusion								31
32 Intravenous Therapy								32
33 Oxygen (Inhalation) Therapy								33
34 Physical Therapy								34
35 Occupational Therapy								35
36 Speech Pathology								36

FORM HCFA-2552-81 (11-81)

19

Exhibit 15 continued

COST ALLOCATION—STATISTICAL BASIS

PROVIDER NO:

WORKSHEET B-1
Continued

37	Electrocardiology	37
38	Electroencephalography	38
39	Medical Supplies Charged to Patients	39
40	Drugs Charged to Patients	40
41	Renal Dialysis	41
42	Kidney Acquisition	42
43		43
44		44
45	**INPATIENT ROUTINE SERVICE COST CENTERS**	45
46	Adults & Pediatrics (General Routine Care)	46
47	Intensive Care Unit	47
48	Coronary Care Unit	48
49		49
50		50
51	Nursery	51
52	Skilled Nursing Facility—Certified	52
53	Skilled Nursing Facility—Noncertified	53
54	**OUTPATIENT SERVICE COST CENTERS**	54
55	Clinic	55
56	Emergency	56
57		57
58	**OTHER REIMBURSABLE COST CENTERS**	58
59	Home Program Dialysis—Other	59
60	Administrative & General—HHA	60
61	Skilled Nursing Care—HHA	61
62	Medical Social Services—HHA	62
63	Home Health Aide—HHA	63
64	Medical Appliances—HHA/DME-Rented	64
65	Durable Medical Equipment Sold	65
66	Home Delivered Meals—HHA	66
67	Other Home Health Services—HHA	67
68	Home Program Dialysis Equipment—100% Medicare	68
69	Ambulance Services	69
70	Intern-Resident Service (not in approved teaching program)	70
71		71
72	SUBTOTALS (Sum of lines 9-71)	72
73	**NONREIMBURSABLE COST CENTERS**	73
74	Gift, Flower, Coffee Shops & Canteen	74
75	Research	75
76	Physicians' Private Offices	76
77	Nonpaid Workers	77
78		78
79	Cost to be Allocated (Per Wkst. B)	79
80	Unit Cost Multiplier	80

FORM HCFA-2552-81 (11-81)

19 continued

Exhibit 15 continued

WORKSHEET B-1

FORM APPROVED
OMB NO. 0938-0050

COST ALLOCATION—STATISTICAL BASIS

PROVIDER NO.

PERIOD:
FROM
TO

	PHARMACY (COSTED REQUISITIONS) 15	MEDICAL RECORDS & LIBRARY (TIME SPENT) 16	SOCIAL SERVICE (TIME SPENT) 17	NURSING SCHOOL (ASSIGNED TIME) 18	INTERN-RESIDENT SERVICE (IN APPROVED TEACHING PROGRAM) (ASSIGNED TIME) 19	20	21
COST CENTER (OMIT CENTS)	$						
1 GENERAL SERVICE COST CENTERS $							
2 Depreciation—Buildings & Fixtures							
3 Depreciation—Movable Equipment							
4 Employee Health & Welfare							
5 Administrative & General							
6 Maintenance & Repairs							
7 Operation of Plant							
8 Laundry & Linen Service							
9 Housekeeping							
10 Dietary							
11 Cafeteria							
12 Maintenance of Personnel							
13 Nursing Administration							
14 Central Services & Supply							
15 Pharmacy	$						
16 Medical Records & Library							
17 Social Service							
18 Nursing School							
19 Intern-Resident Service (in approved teaching program)							
20							
21 ANCILLARY SERVICE COST CENTERS							
22 Operating Room							
23 Recovery Room							
24 Delivery Room & Labor Room							
25 Anesthesiology							
26 Radiology—Diagnostic							
27 Radiology—Therapeutic							
28 Radioisotope							
29 Laboratory							
30 Whole Blood and Packed Red Blood Cells							
31 Blood Storing, Processing and Transfusion							
32 Intravenous Therapy							
33 Oxygen (Inhalation) Therapy							
34 Physical Therapy							
35 Occupational Therapy							
36 Speech Pathology							

FORM HCFA-2552-81 (11-81)

Exhibit 15 continued

COST ALLOCATION—STATISTICAL BASIS

PROVIDER NO

WORKSHEET B-1
Continued

37	Electrocardiology
38	Electroencephalography
39	Medical Supplies Charged to Patients
40	Drugs Charged to Patients
41	Renal Dialysis
42	Kidney Acquisition
43	
44	
45	INPATIENT ROUTINE SERVICE COST CENTERS
46	Adults & Pediatrics (General Routine Care)
47	Intensive Care Unit
48	Coronary Care Unit
49	
50	
51	Nursery
52	Skilled Nursing Facility—Certified
53	Skilled Nursing Facility—Noncertified
54	OUTPATIENT SERVICE COST CENTERS
55	Clinic
56	Emergency
57	
58	OTHER REIMBURSABLE COST CENTERS
59	Home Program Dialysis—Other
60	Administrative & General—HHA
61	Skilled Nursing Care—HHA
62	Medical Social Services—HHA
63	Home Health Aide—HHA
64	Medical Appliances—HHA/DME-Rented
65	Durable Medical Equipment Sold
66	Home Delivered Meals—HHA
67	Other Home Health Services—HHA
68	Home Program Dialysis Equipment—100% Medicare
69	Ambulance Services
70	Intern-Resident Service (not in approved teaching program)
71	
72	SUBTOTALS (Sum of lines 16-71)
73	NONREIMBURSABLE COST CENTERS
74	Gift, Flower, Coffee Shops & Canteen
75	Research
76	Physicians' Private Offices
77	Nonpaid Workers
78	
79	Cost to be Allocated (Per Wkst. B)
80	Unit Cost Multiple

FORM HCFA-2552-81 (11-81)

20 continued

Appendix D

Medicare Regulations Regarding Hospital Revenue and Pricing Strategies

The following Medicare instructions apply, at this writing, to the use of hospital revenue and pricing strategies, as discussed in Chapter 6. Relevant worksheets, identified by exhibit number from the list of worksheets in Appendix F, follow the instructions. Pricing strategy techniques are applied on Medicare Worksheet C and Worksheet D.

supporting worksheet showing the computation of the amounts entered
on Worksheet B-1, column 5, lines 6 through 73. That cost,
which was reduced by the grant, must be fully reflected in the
appropriate cost center(s) in this column to receive a fair
share of administrative and general expense.

A negative cost center balance in the statistics for allocating
administrative and general expenses causes an improper distribution of this overhead cost center. Negative balances must be
excluded from the allocation statistics when administrative and
general expenses are allocated on the basis of accumulated cost.

On the other hand, in arriving at the amounts entered in the
subtotal column of Worksheet B before allocation of administrative
and general expenses (column 4a) some cost centers may have
negative balances caused by offsets of grants, gifts or endowment
income. In this situation, the full amount of such offsets to
these cost centers is restored to the balances before they are
entered on Worksheet B-1, column 5, as allocation statistics for
the administrative and general cost center. After the restoration
of offsets due to grants, gifts and endowment income, and there
is still a negative balance, exclude the negative balance from
the allocation statistics when the administrative and general
expenses are allocated on the basis of accumulated cost.

330. WORKSHEET C - DEPARTMENTAL COST DISTRIBUTION
On this worksheet the lines in column 1 and columns 3 through 10
are divided by a dotted rule into two parts: Part a and Part b.
In each instance, cost data is entered in Part b.

THE PROVIDER SHOULD SUBMIT ALL DATA REQUESTED IN COLUMNS 1 THROUGH
10, LINES 1 THROUGH 33, AS APPROPRIATE.

Column 1--Enter on Part a of each line, the total cost of each cost
center as computed on Worksheet B, column 21, lines 22 through
41, 43 and 44, 55 through 57 and 59 through 63. Exceptions:
(1) When adjustments to expenses are required after cost allocation
(e.g., adjustments needed for allocation of standby costs or
adjustments for costs applicable to unoccupied beds of a provider
with a restrictive admission policy), the adjusted cost center
expenses to be entered on Worksheet C must be obtained from the
supporting worksheet submitted by the provider. See the instructions for completing Worksheet B; (2) Providers that furnish
outpatient renal dialysis services and use either an inpatient
routine bed, or a bed or other accommodation in the outpatient area
(other than in the renal dialysis department) to furnish this
service must adjust the renal dialysis cost computed on
Worksheet B, column 21, line 41. In this instance, adjusted renal
dialysis cost to be entered on line 21a is obtained from
Supplemental Worksheet D-7, Part III, line 3; (3) Any cost center
with a credit balance is not brought forward from Worksheet B,

column 21. However, the charges applicable to such cost centers
with a credit balance must be reported on Part b of the appropriate
line on Worksheet C.

Enter on Part b of each line (from the provider's records) the
total gross charges for all patients for each cost center. The
charges for all departments using combined billing should be
either gross combined charges for professional and provider
components or gross charges for provider component only. If
gross combined charges are used, gross combined charges must be
used on Worksheet D to apportion inpatient ancillary service
costs to the health care programs and on Worksheet D-3 to apportion the physician remuneration for professional services under
combined billing to the health care programs. If gross charges
for the provider component only are used, gross charges for the
provider component only must be used on Worksheet D to apportion
inpatient ancillary service costs to the health care programs,
and gross charges for the professional component only must be
used on Worksheet D-3 to apportion the physician remuneration
for professional services under combined billing to the program.

When certain services are furnished under arrangements and an
adjustment was made on Worksheet A-8 to "gross up" costs, the
related charges entered on Worksheet C must also be "grossed up"
in accordance with PRM, Part I, chapter 23.

NOTE: The standard charges of the renal dialysis cost center
       should have been developed to properly reflect the total
       cost of furnishing renal dialysis, including the cost
       transferred from the inpatient routine areas and the
       outpatient departments.

Column 2--Divide the cost on Part a of each line in column 1 by
charges on Part b of each line in column 1 to determine the ratio
of total cost to total charges for each cost center. Enter the
resultant departmental ratios in column 2.

Columns 3 through 10--For each provider component or each patient
classification, as listed in the column headings, enter the gross
departmental charges - all patients (Skilled Nursing Facility -
Certified in column 6), (title XVIII - Part B outpatient charges
in column 7 and Kidney Acquisition charges in column 8) on Part b
of each line (lines 2-33).

The charges applicable to the noncertified portion of a skilled
nursing facility should be entered in column 4 or column 5, if
either of these columns are not being used to record charges
applicable to a subprovider. If both column 4 and column 5 are
not available, the provider should enter the data relative to
the noncertified portion of the skilled nursing facility on a
separate Worksheet C. For each line, multiply the charges on

Part b by the departmental ratios in column 2 (same line) to
determine the departmental cost, which is to be entered in the
appropriate columns on Part a of each line.

Enter on line 34a, the sum of lines 2a through 33a. Enter on
line 34b, the sum of lines 2b through 33b.

NOTE: Column 8 (Kidney Acquisition) will not be completed when
        the provider elects to be reimbursed for kidney acqui-
        sition costs under the ALTERNATIVE PROCEDURES as explained
        in the instructions to Supplemental Worksheet D-6
        (Computation of Kidney Acquisition Costs and Charges -
        Supplementary to Inpatient Routine and Inpatient Ancillary
        Service Costs and Charges). If the provider has elected to
        be reimbursed under the ALTERNATIVE PROCEDURES, the kidney
        acquisition outpatient charges should be included in
        inpatient charges of the hospital (column 3) and be
        excluded from outpatient charges.

Transfer the amounts on this worksheet as follows:

        1. Because the target rate reimbursement option is
available for home program dialysis services, the Part B, title
XVIII outpatient costs in column 7 will be transferred as follows:

        a. Target Rate Reimbursement Elected - Transfer the
amount on line 34a minus the amount on line 29a to Worksheet E,
Part I, column 2, line 2.

        b. Cost Reimbursement - Transfer the amount on
line 34a to Worksheet E, Part I, column 2, line 2.

        2. Transfer the kidney acquisition costs in column 8,
line 34a to Supplemental Worksheet D-6, Part I, line 3.

        3. Transfer the home health agency costs in column 10,
line 34a to form HCFA-1728A for cost reporting periods beginning on
or after July 1, 1979, and to form HCFA-1729 for cost reporting
periods beginning on or after October 1, 1980.

332. WORKSHEET D - APPORTIONMENT OF INPATIENT ANCILLARY SERVICES TO
      HEALTH CARE PROGRAMS
A separate copy of this worksheet must be completed for the hospital,
skilled nursing facility, each subprovider and hospital-based
skilled nursing facility.

Column 1--Enter the ratio of cost to charges developed for each
cost center on Worksheet C, column 2.

Columns 2 through 5--Enter from the provider's records, the
appropriate health care program inpatient charges for the indicated cost centers. If gross combined charges for professional

3-52   Rev. 8-80 and provider components were used on Worksheet C to determine the ratio entered in column 1, then gross combined charges applicable to each health care program should be entered in columns 2 through 5, as appropriate. If gross charges for provider component only were used, then only the health care program gross charges for provider component should be used in columns 2 through 5, as appropriate.

NOTE: All hospital inpatient ancillary service charges applicable to living and cadaveric kidney donors (whether the kidney recipient is Medicare or non-Medicare) should be included in title XVIII - Part A inpatient charges. As such, the inpatient ancillary cost applicable to all kidney acquisitions is apportioned to and included in title XVIII - Part A inpatient ancillary costs. Also, the charges generated in the rendition of kidney acquisition hospital outpatient services should be included with title XVIII - Part A inpatient charges and omitted from outpatient charges, the same as the treatment being afforded hospital inpatient ancillary kidney acquisition charges, whenever the provider has elected to be reimbursed for kidney acquisition costs under the ALTERNATIVE PROCEDURES as explained in the instructions to Supplemental Worksheet D-6 (Computation of Kidney Acquisition Costs and Charges - Supplementary to Inpatient Routine and Inpatient Ancillary Service Cost and Charges).

Columns 6 through 9—Multiply the indicated health care program inpatient charges in columns 2 through 5 by the ratio in column 1 to determine the health care program inpatient expenses.

334. WORKSHEET D-1 - COMPUTATION OF INPATIENT ROUTINE SERVICE COST
This worksheet provides for the apportionment of inpatient routine service costs to the health care programs. Where applicable, provision is also made for the computation of the inpatient routine nursing salary cost differential. In addition, this worksheet provides for the computation of the reasonable cost limitation for general inpatient routine care. This worksheet consists of two parts - Part I for title XVIII (Medicare) and Part II for titles V and XIX. A separate copy of Part II must be completed for title V and title XIX.

The average per diem computations on this worksheet must be rounded to two decimal places (92,848 divided by 1000 days = $92.848, rounded to $92.85).

INPATIENT ROUTINE NURSING SALARY COST DIFFERENTIAL
An inpatient routine nursing salary cost differential is applicable as an element in the computation of the provider's reimbursable cost. For skilled nursing facilities, the inpatient routine nursing salary cost differential rate is 8½ percent. For hospitals and subproviders, the inpatient routine nursing salary cost differential rate in effect until September 30, 1981, is 8½ percent. As of October 1, 1981, the rate for hospitals and subproviders is changed to 5 percent.

For hospital and subprovider cost reporting periods beginning before October 1, 1981, and ending after September 30, 1981, the 8½ percent rate is applicable for that portion of the cost reporting period occurring before October 1, 1981, and the 5 percent rate is applicable for that portion of the cost reporting period occurring after September 30, 1981.

For hospital and subprovider cost reporting periods which include 12 full calendar months and which end on the last day of a month, a composite nursing differential percentage will be used. This composite is based on the number of months in the reporting period occurring prior to October 1, 1981, and the number of months ending after September 30, 1981. Under these conditions, the following table will be used to compute the routine nursing salary cost differential:

12-Month Cost Reporting Period Ending Date	Nursing Differential Percentage
October 31, 1981	1.082
November 30, 1981	1.080
December 31, 1981	1.077
January 31, 1982	1.074
February 28, 1982	1.071
March 31, 1982	1.068
April 30, 1982	1.065
May 31, 1982	1.062
June 30, 1982	1.059
July 31, 1982	1.056
August 31, 1982	1.053
September 30, 1982 and there-after	1.05

For hospital and subprovider cost reporting periods ending on a day other than on the last day of the month, or for cost reporting periods of less than 12 months, an appropriate aggregate percentage should be developed using the following formula:

$$\frac{(A \times 1.085) + (B \times 1.05)}{C} = NDP$$

A = Total days in the cost reporting period prior to 10/1/81.
B = Total days in the cost reporting period after 9/30/81.
C = Total number of days (A) plus (B).
NDP = Nursing Differential Percentage.

The nursing differential percentage must be rounded to three decimal places.

Exhibit 16

FORM APPROVED
OMB NO. 0938-0050

WORKSHEET C

DEPARTMENTAL COST DISTRIBUTION

PROVIDER NO. _____

PERIOD FROM _____ TO _____

COST CENTER	TOTAL (From Wkst. B, Col. 21)	RATIO OF COST TO CHARGES	HOSPITAL (COL. 2 X 3b)	SUBPROVIDER I (COL. 2 X 4b)	SUBPROVIDER II (COL. 2 X 5b)	SKILLED NURSING FACILITY—CERTIFIED (COL. 2 X 6b)	PART B HHA (COL. 2 X 7b)	PART B OUTPATIENT EMERGENCY SERVICE (COL. 2 X 8b)
	1	2	3	4	5	6	7	8
1 ANCILLARY SERVICE COST CENTERS								
2 Operating Room								
3 Recovery Room								
4 Delivery Room & Labor Room								
5 Anesthesiology								
6 Radiology—Diagnostic								
7 Radiology—Therapeutic								
8 Radioisotope								
9 Laboratory								
10 Whole Blood and Packed Red Blood Cells								
11 Blood Storing, Processing & Transfusion								
12 Intravenous Therapy								
13 Oxygen (Inhalation) Therapy								
14 Physical Therapy								
15 Occupational Therapy								
16 Speech Pathology								
17 Electrocardiology								
18 Electroencephalography								

FORM HCFA-2552-81 (11-81)

Exhibit 16 continued

WORKSHEET C
Continued

PROVIDER NO.

DEPARTMENTAL COST DISTRIBUTION

		1	2	3	4	5	6	7	8	
19	Medical Supplies Charged to Patients									19
20	Drugs Charged to Patients									20
21	Renal Dialysis									21
22										22
23										23
24	OUTPATIENT SERVICE COST CENTERS									24
25	Clinic									25
26	Emergency									26
27										27
28	OTHER REIMBURSABLE COST CENTERS									28
29	Home Program Dialysis—Other									29
30	TOTAL									30

21 Continued

FORM HCFA-2552-81 (11-81)

Exhibit 16 continued

DEPARTMENTAL COST DISTRIBUTION

WORKSHEET C

PROVIDER NO

PERIOD FROM ___ TO ___

COST CENTER		RATIO OF COST TO CHARGES (2)	TITLE XVIII OUTPATIENT			OTHER OUTPATIENT				HOME HEALTH AGENCY (COL. 2 × 15b) (15)	
			RENAL DIALYSIS (COL. 2 × 9b) (9)	PART B ALL OTHER (COL. 7 × 10b) (10)	KIDNEY ACQUISITION (COL. 2 × 11b) (11)	RENAL DIALYSIS (COL. 2 × 12b) (12)	MEDICAL EMERGENCY (COL. 2 × 13b) (13)	ALL OTHER OUTPATIENT (COL. 2 × 14b) (14)			
1	ANCILLARY SERVICE COST CENTERS										1
2	Operating Room	a / b		$			$	$			2
3	Recovery Room	a / b		$			$	$			3
4	Delivery Room & Labor Room	a / b		$			$	$			4
5	Anesthesiology	a / b		$	$		$	$			5
6	Radiology—Diagnostic	a / b		$	$		$	$			6
7	Radiology—Therapeutic	a / b		$	$		$	$			7
8	Radioisotope	a / b		$	$		$	$			8
9	Laboratory	a / b	$	$	$	$	$	$			9
10	Whole Blood and Packed Red Blood Cells	a / b		$	$		$	$			10
11	Blood Storing, Processing and Transfusion	a / b		$	$		$	$			11
12	Intravenous Therapy	a / b		$			$	$			12
13	Oxygen (Inhalation) Therapy	a / b	$	$		$	$	$			13
14	Physical Therapy	a / b		$			$	$	$		14
15	Occupational Therapy	a / b		$			$	$	$		15
16	Speech Pathology	a / b		$			$	$	$		16
17	Electrocardiology	a / b		$	$		$	$			17
18	Electroencephalography	a / b		$	$		$	$			18

22

FORM HCFA-2552-81 (11-81)

Exhibit 16 continued

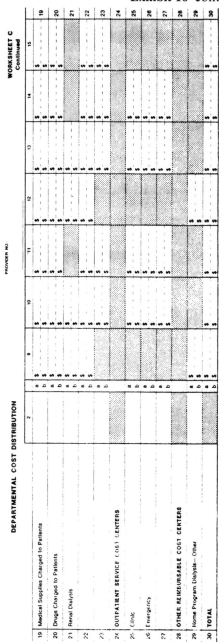

Exhibit 17

FORM APPROVED
OMB NO. 0938-0050

WORKSHEET D

APPORTIONMENT OF INPATIENT ANCILLARY SERVICES TO HEALTH CARE PROGRAMS

CHECK ONE ☐ HOSPITAL   ☐ SUBPROVIDER I   ☐ SUBPROVIDER II   ☐ SKILLED NURSING FACILITY

PROVIDER NO _____   PERIOD FROM _____ TO _____

COST CENTER	RATIO OF COST TO CHARGES (FR. WKST C, COL 2)	TITLE V	HEALTH CARE PROGRAM INPATIENT CHARGES		TITLE XIX	TITLE V (1) (COL 1 × COL 2)	HEALTH CARE PROGRAM INPATIENT EXPENSES			
			TITLE XVIII PART A	PART B			TITLE XVIII (2) PART A (COL 1 × COL 3)	PART B (COL 1 × COL 4)	TITLE XIX (1) (COL 1 × COL 5)	
	1	2	3	4	5	6	7	8	9	
ANCILLARY SERVICE COST CENTERS										1
Operating Room		$			$	$	$	$	$	2
Recovery Room										3
Delivery Room & Labor Room										4
Anesthesiology										5
Radiology—Diagnostic										6
Radiology—Therapeutic			$					$		7
Radioisotope										8
Laboratory										9
Whole Blood and Packed Red Blood Cells										10
Blood Storing, Processing and Transfusion										11
Intravenous Therapy										12
Oxygen (Inhalation) Therapy										13
Physical Therapy										14
Occupational Therapy										15
Speech Pathology										16
Electrocardiology										17
Electroencephalography										18
Medical Supplies Charged to Patients										19
Drugs Charged to Patients										20
Renal Dialysis										21
										22
										23
OUTPATIENT SERVICE COST CENTERS										24
Clinic										25
Emergency										26
										27
TOTAL		$	$	$	$	$	$	$	$	28

(1) Transfer the amounts in column 6 and column 9, line 28, to the appropriate Worksheet E-5, Part I, column as appropriate, line 1.
(2) Transfer the amounts in column 7 and column 8, line 28, to Worksheet E, Part I, column as appropriate, line 1.

23

FORM HCFA-2552-81 (11-81)

Medicare Regulations Regarding the Hospital Cost Apportionment Process

The following Medicare instructions apply, at this writing, to the hospital cost apportionment process, as discussed in Chapter 7. Relevant worksheets, identified by exhibit number from the list of worksheets in Appendix F, follow the instructions. Apportionment techniques are applied on Medicare Worksheet D-1 through Worksheet D-6.

The nursing differential percentage for hospitals and subproviders will be used in Part I, lines 4 and 12, in place of the 1.085 percent printed on the form. For skilled nursing facilities (including provider-based skilled nursing facilities), continue to use 1.085 as indicated on the form.

334.1   Part I - Title XVIII (Medicare).—This part consists of two sections - General Inpatient Care Units (including provisions for inpatient routine nursing salary cost differential, reasonable cost limitation and the capital-related cost and educational cost exclusions) and intensive care type inpatient hospital units.

GENERAL INPATIENT CARE UNITS (LINES 1 THROUGH 39)
With the exception of providers that have only aged, pediatric and maternity patients, or that have only patients other than aged, pediatric and maternity, providers must complete all of these lines. Providers having only aged, pediatric and maternity patients or only patients other than aged, pediatric and maternity, so that the inpatient routine nursing salary cost differential does not apply, should complete lines 3, 8, 11, 19 and 22 through 39. For such providers, the instruction for line 19 should be changed to read "(line 11 divided by line 3)," and the instruction for line 22 should be changed to read "(line 19 x line 8)."

NOTE: Do not include any inpatient days or costs applicable to intensive care, coronary care or other intensive care type inpatient hospital units. They should be included on lines 40 through 43.

LINE DESCRIPTIONS

Line 4—For hospital and subprovider cost reports, multiply the aged, pediatric and maternity days on line 1 by the nursing differential percentage applicable to your fiscal year as determined above.

For skilled nursing facility cost reports (including provider-based skilled nursing facilities), multiply the aged, pediatric and maternity days on line 1 by 1.085. This has the effect of increasing these days by 8] percent, for the purpose of computing the inpatient routine nursing salary cost differential.

Lines 6-8—Enter the total Medicare inpatient days on line 8, detailed by Medicare aged, pediatric and maternity days on line 6 and Medicare inpatient days other than aged, pediatric and maternity days on line 7.

NOTE: Inpatient days applicable to outpatient renal dialysis must not be included in Medicare days. However, inpatient days applicable to outpatient renal dialysis must be included in the total inpatient day count on lines 1, 2 and 3.

The computation of inpatient days applicable to outpatient renal dialysis is applicable only where providers use inpatient beds (rather than beds in the dialysis department) in furnishing outpatient renal dialysis (either hemodialysis or peritoneal dialysis) services.

Line 9—Enter the total inpatient routine nursing salary cost. The nursing salary cost includable on this line is defined in HCFA Pub. 15-I, chapter 13, and must be obtained from the provider's records.

Line 10—Enter the balance of the total allowable inpatient routine service cost which excludes the inpatient routine nursing salary cost entered on line 9.

Line 11—The total general inpatient routine service cost on this line must agree with the following amounts on Worksheet B, column 21:

> Hospital - line 46
> Subprovider I - line 49 or line 50
> Subprovider II - line 49 or line 50
> Skilled Nursing Facility - Certified - line 52

Line 12—For hospital and subprovider cost reports, multiply the total inpatient routine nursing salary cost on line 9 by the same nursing differential percentage which was used on line 4 above.

For skilled nursing facility (including provider-based skilled nursing facility) cost reports, multiply the inpatient routine nursing salary cost on line 9 by 1.085. This has the effect of increasing this cost by 8½ percent and is used to compute the inpatient routine nursing salary cost differential.

Lines 13-19—Compute the adjusted average per diem general inpatient routine service cost applicable to all aged, pediatric and maternity patients, and the average per diem general inpatient routine service cost applicable to all patients other than aged, pediatric and maternity in accordance with the insert captions shown on each of these lines.

Lines 20-22—Compute the total Medicare general inpatient routine service cost in accordance with the insert captions shown on these lines.

Line 23—Enter on this line the provider charges to beneficiaries for excess costs as determined in accordance with HCFA Pub. 15-I, chapter 25. Any amounts erroneously collected (based on a subsequently raised cost limit) from the beneficiaries for excess costs should be excluded from the amount entered on line 23.

Line 24—Subtract line 23 from line 22 and enter the difference.

NOTE: New providers are not subject to the reasonable cost limitation and, therefore,
        do not complete lines 25 through 38. The amount on line 24 is transferred directly
        to line 39. A "new provider" is an institution that has operated as the type of
        facility (or equivalent thereof) for which it is certified in the program under
        present and previous ownership for less than 3 full years. (See Health Insurance
        regulations section 405.460.)

Lines 25-28—These lines are provided to compute the amount of allocated capital-related
costs that are part of the general inpatient routine service cost. The format and allocation
process to be employed is identical to that used on Worksheets B and B-1. Only the
general service cost centers and the general inpatient routine service cost centers are
displayed because they are the cost centers needed in determining the capital-related
cost applicable to general inpatient routine service cost centers. Lines 25.4 to 25.52
and 26.4 to 26.52 and columns 4 through 21 are identical to the lines and columns on
Worksheets B and B-1.

The amounts to be entered in column 1, lines 25.4 to 25.52 are obtained from Worksheet
B, column 2, lines 4 through 20, 46, 49, 50 and 52. The amounts to be entered in column
2, lines 25.4 to 25.52 are obtained from Worksheet B, column 3, lines 4 through 20, 46,
49, 50 and 52. Where providers have directly assigned capital-related costs, enter those
amounts from the provider's records.

The statistics for allocating capital-related costs will be displayed on lines 26.4 to 26.52.
The statistics are obtained from Worksheet B-1, columns as appropriate, lines 4 through
20, 46, 49, 50 and 52. Enter on the first line in the column of the cost center being
allocated, the total statistical base over which the expenses are to be allocated (e.g.,
column 4 - Employee Health and Welfare, enter on line 26.4, the total statistics from
Worksheet B-1, column 4, line 4; enter on line 26.5, the statistics from Worksheet B-
1, column 4, line 5, etc.). The allocation process is identical to that used on Worksheets
B and B-1.

Lines 25.AA and 26.AA are used to accumulate the costs and statistics applicable to
the remainder of the cost center (ancillary, intensive care type inpatient hospital units,
nursery, SNF-noncertified, outpatient, other reimbursable and nonreimbursable) on Worksheets
B and B-1. Note that for the shaded areas in columns 18 and 19 on this worksheet, the
costs and statistics applicable to those shaded areas are included with "other" accumulated
amounts on lines 25.AA and 26.AA, as appropriate.

EXCEPTION: When a general service cost center is not allocated on Worksheet B because
           it has a credit balance at the point it would normally be allocated, the capital-
           related costs for the same general service cost center should be entered on line
           25.AA. The total statistics applicable to such cost center with a credit balance
           should be entered on line 26.AA as well as on the first line of the cost center
           being allocated.

Also, when a general service cost center has a negative direct expense balance on Worksheet B, column 1, and the negative balance becomes a positive balance through the cost allocation process, the amount of capital-related costs determined on line 25 for that general service cost center must be adjusted to reflect the amount that was allocated on Worksheet B. The adjusted amount of capital-related costs to be allocated on line 25 is computed by dividing the capital-related costs determined on line 25 by the total indirect cost allocated to the cost center on Worksheet B (do not include the negative direct expenses) and multiplying that ratio times the net amount allocated on Worksheet B for that cost center.

For example: The net expenses for cost allocation on Worksheet B, column 1, line 11 (Cafeteria) is a negative $45,000. After other general service cost centers have been allocated to the Cafeteria cost center, the amount of Cafeteria costs to be allocated on Worksheet B, column 11, line 11, is a positive $29,650. The total overhead allocated to Cafeteria on Worksheet B is $74,650 ($45,000 plus $29,650). The total amount of capital-related costs allocated to the Cafeteria cost center on Worksheet D-1, column 11, line 25.11 is $24,774. However, the actual amount of capital-related costs for the Cafeteria cost center to be allocated on Worksheet D-1, column 11, line 25.11 must equal the actual amount which was allocated on Worksheet B, column 11, line 11 and is computed as follows: $24,774 divided by $74,650 = .33186872 times $29,650 = $9,840. Therefore, $9,840 will be the amount of capital-related costs to be allocated on Worksheet D-1, column 11, line 25.11 for the Cafeteria cost center. Enter the amount of this adjustment on line 25.AB so that line 25 will crossfoot.

Enter on line 27 the total capital-related costs of the cost center to be allocated. This amount is obtained from line 25, from the first line of the column being allocated (e.g., in the case of Employee Health and Welfare, the amount to be entered in column 4, line 27, is obtained from column 4, line 25.4).

Divide the amount entered on line 27 by the total statistical base entered in the same column on the first subline of line 26. Enter the resulting Unit Cost Multiplier on line 28. The Unit Cost Multiplier shown must be at least eight decimal places. The Unit Cost Multipliers must be different than those on Worksheet B-1 because only a portion of the total which was allocated on Worksheet B is being allocated on line 25.

Multiply that portion of the total statistical base applicable to each cost center receiving the capital-related costs by the Unit Cost Multiplier. Enter on line 25 in the corresponding column and line, the result of each computation on line 26.

After all the capital-related costs of the general service cost centers have been allocated on line 25, enter in column 21, the sum of columns 3 through 20, for lines 25.46, 25.49, 25.50 and 25.52. These amounts represent the capital-related costs which are excluded from general inpatient routine costs before the application of the cost limit. Columns 18 and 19 for the hospital and subproviders are shaded because the full amount of educational costs are obtained from Worksheet B, columns 18 and 19, lines 46, 49 and 50. See the insert reference on this worksheet, line 30.

Transfer the total amounts in column 21, lines 25.46, 25.49, 25.50 and 25.52 to line 29 as follows:

From line 25.46 to line 29, column 1 (hospital)
From line 25.49 to line 29, column 2 (subprovider)
From line 25.50 to line 29, column 3 (subprovider)
From line 25.52 to line 29, column 4 (skilled nursing facility)

Line 35—Enter on this line the general inpatient routine service cost limitation which is determined by multiplying the number of Medicare inpatient days on line 8 by the cost limit for general inpatient routine service cost applicable to the provider for the period for which the cost report is being filed.

Hospitals and subproviders with cost reporting periods beginning before October 1, 1981, and ending after September 30, 1981, will be governed by two schedules of cost limits: (1) the schedule in effect on the first day of the reporting period which will be applied in proportion to the part of the total period occurring between the first day of the period and ending September 30, 1981, and (2) the schedule in effect which will be applied in proportion to the part of the total period occurring after September 30, 1981. Two alternatives for calculating the application of the cost limits are provided in the example below. A supporting worksheet showing the complete computation of the total allowable cost must be attached to Worksheet D-1 based on the examples provided below.

Example 1   A hospital has a cost reporting period which begins December 1, 1980. Assume that the hospital's limit for this period is $177.24, and the limit for that portion of the period ending after September 30, 1981, is $170.24. Assume also that hospital had 1,000 general routine patient days during the entire cost reporting period.

It is first necessary to determine what total allowable cost would be for the entire period under both the old and new limits (even though neither the old nor the new limit, in fact, applies to the entire period). This is done as follows:

Total allowable cost for the entire period using old limit:

$177.24 X 1,000 days = $177,240

Total allowable cost for the entire period using new limit:

$170.24 X 1,000 days = $170,240

Difference = $7,000

It is then necessary to determine what proportion of this difference should be applied to the months after September 30, 1981. This is accomplished as follows:

$7,000 X 2/12 (number of months after 9-30-81 in the hospital's cost reporting period) = $1,167

To determine the actual total allowable cost, the amount of the disallowance under the new limits ($1,167) is subtracted from the total allowable costs for the entire period (under the old limit) as follows:

Total allowable cost for the period:	$177,240
	−1,167
	$176,073

Example 2: Assume the same facts as in example 1.

Total allowable costs for the entire period using old limit: $177,240.

Ratio of new limit to old limit $170.24 to $177.24 is .96050.

.96050 represents the proportion which the new limit bears to the old limit. However, since the new limit applies only to months in the reporting period after September 30, 1981, it is necessary to increase this proportion to reflect this fact. This is done by the formula below. .0395 represents the total percentage reduction in the new limit (1.00 − .96050). This figure is then reduced in proportion to the number of months subject to the old limit (10), and the result is added to .96050 to obtain the relationship which total allowable costs using the proportional application of the new limits bears to total allowable costs computed under the old limits for the entire period.

((.0395 X 10 divided by 12) + .96050) X $177,240 = $176,073—Total allowable cost for the period.

Line 36—Enter on this line the amount which is determined by multiplying the number of living and cadaveric donor kidney acquisition days by the per diem charge otherwise billable to beneficiaries for excess provider costs.

NOTE: No amount should be entered on this line if no entry is made on line 23 because the provider has not elected to charge beneficiaries for excess costs.

INTENSIVE CARE TYPE INPATIENT HOSPITAL UNITS (EXCLUDING NURSERY) (LINES 40-43)—These lines provide for the apportionment of the hospital inpatient routine service cost of intensive care type inpatient hospital units (excluding nursery) to the Medicare program. Note that the inpatient routine nursing salary cost differential does not apply to intensive care type inpatient hospital units.

Column 1—Enter on the appropriate line the total inpatient routine cost applicable to each of the indicated intensive care type inpatient hospital units from Worksheet B, column 21, lines 47 through 50, as appropriate.

Column 2—Enter on the appropriate line the total inpatient days applicable to each of the indicated intensive care type inpatient hospital units. These inpatient days must be obtained from the appropriate column on page 2, Part II, line 6.

Column 3—For each line, divide the total inpatient cost in column 1 by the total inpatient days in column 2.

Column 4—Enter on the appropriate line the total Medicare days applicable to each of the indicated intensive care type inpatient hospital units. These inpatient days must be obtained from the appropriate column on page 2, Part II, line 10i.

Column 5—Multiply the average per diem cost in column 3 by the Medicare days in column 4.

Line 44—Enter the sum of the amounts on lines 39 through 43.

Inpatient routine service costs computed on this worksheet must be transferred to Worksheet E, Part I, line 3.

334.2 Part II - Titles V and XIX.--This part provides for the
apportionment of the inpatient routine service costs of general
patient care units, special care units and nursery to titles V
and XIX. A separate copy of this part must be completed for
title V and title XIX.

LINE DESCRIPTIONS

Lines 45-53--These lines provide for the computation of the
average per diem inpatient routine service cost for general
inpatient care units for cost apportionment under titles V and
XIX. Hospitals in which the inpatient routine nursing salary
cost differential under title XVIII does not apply, should not
complete lines 45-52. Instead, enter on line 53, the amount
appearing in Part I, line 19.

Lines 54-56--These lines provide for the computation of the
nursery average per diem cost. Enter on line 54, the amount
from Worksheet B, column 21, line 51. The total newborn days
are obtained from the appropriate column of page 2, Part II,
line 8, or page 3, Part IV, line 8.

Lines 57 and 58--Compute the total general inpatient routine
service cost applicable to titles V and XIX before reasonable
cost limitations in accordance with the insert captions shown on
these lines.

Lines 59-62--These lines provide for the application of the
reasonable cost limitation and the computation of reimbursable
general inpatient routine service cost. See the instructions for
lines 23 through 39 for an explanation of these lines. NOTE:
Lines 23, 36 and 37 are not applicable under titles V and XIX.

Lines 63-67--These lines provide for the computation of the
remaining inpatient routine service costs applicable to titles V
and XIX. The days in column 1, line 63, are obtained from page 2,
Part II, column 1, line 9b for title V or line 11b for title XIX;
or the appropriate column of page 3, Part IV, line 9b for
title V or line 11b for title XIX. The days in column 1, lines 64
through 67 are obtained from the appropriate column of page 2,
Part II, line 9a for title V or line 11a for title XIX.

Line 68--Enter the sum of the amounts on lines 62 through 67.
Transfer the totals to the appropriate columns on the appropriate
Worksheet E-5, Part I, line 2.

336. WORKSHEET D-2 - APPORTIONMENT OF COST OF SERVICES RENDERED
      BY INTERNS AND RESIDENTS

336.1 Part I - Not in Approved Teaching Program.--This part is to
be used only by providers having interns and residents who are not
in an approved teaching program. (See PRM, Part I, chapter 4.)

Column 1--Enter the percentage of time that interns and residents are assigned to each of the indicated patient care areas.

Column 2--Enter on line 1, the total cost of services rendered in all patient care areas from Worksheet B, column 21, line 66. Multiply each of the percentages in column 1 by the total cost in column 2, line 1. Enter the resulting amounts on the appropriate lines in column 2.

Column 3--The total inpatient days applicable to the various patient care areas of the complex and entered in column 3 must agree with the total inpatient days for each patient care area shown on page 2, Part II, lines 6 and 8, or on page 3, Part IV, lines 6 and 8, as appropriate.

Column 4--Divide the allocated expense in column 2 by the inpatient days in column 3 to arrive at the average per diem cost.

Columns 5, 6 and 7--Enter in the appropriate column the health care program inpatient days for each patient care area:

> Title V--Page 2, Part II, lines 9a and 9b, or page 3, Part IV, lines 9a and 9b, as appropriate.

> Title XVIII--Page 2, Part II, line 10j, or page 3, Part IV, line 10j, as appropriate.

NOTE: If the provider has elected to be reimbursed for kidney acquisition costs under the ALTERNATIVE PROCEDURES (see the instructions for completing Supplemental Worksheet D-6), the days in column 6 will be the sum of page 2, Part II, lines 10h and 10j, or page 3, Part IV, lines 10h and 10j, as appropriate.

> Title XIX--Page 2, Part II, lines 11a and 11b, or page 3, Part IV, lines 11a and 11b, as appropriate.

Columns 8, 9 and 10--Multiply the average cost per day in column 4 by the health care program days in columns 5, 6 and 7, respectively. Enter the resulting amounts in columns 8, 9, and 10, as appropriate.

Columns a, b, c, d and e--These columns provide for computing the ratio of total expenses in each of the hospital outpatient service areas to total charges in each of the hospital outpatient service areas. These ratios are the basis for apportioning to Medicare its share of the cost of intern and resident services applicable to hospital outpatient services. Accordingly, multiply the amounts shown in column d by the ratios developed in column e. Enter the resulting amounts in column 9.

The expenses entered on lines 9, 10 and 11, applicable to
title V (column 8) and title XIX (column 10), are transferred to
Worksheet E-5, Part I, column as appropriate, line 3. The expenses
entered in column 9, lines 9, 10, 11, 12 and 20 should be transferred to the appropriate lines in Part III, column 2, whenever
both Parts I and II are completed. However, when only Part I is
completed, the sum of the amounts entered in column 9 on lines 9
and 20 and the amounts entered on lines 10, 11 and 12, applicable
to title XVIII, are transferred directly to Worksheet E, Part I,
columns 2, 4, 6 and 8, as appropriate, line 4.

336.2 Part II - In an Approved Teaching Program (Part B Inpatient
Routine Costs Only).--This part provides for reimbursement for
inpatient routine services which are rendered by interns and
residents in approved teaching programs to Medicare beneficiaries
who have Part B coverage and who have exhausted or are not
entitled to benefits under Part A. (See PRM, Part I, chapters 4
and 21.)

Column 1--Enter the amounts allocated in the cost-finding process
to the indicated cost centers. These amounts are obtained from
Worksheet B, column 19.

Column 2--The total inpatient days applicable to the various
patient care areas of the complex and to be entered in column 2
must agree with the total inpatient days for each patient care
area on page 2, Part II, line 6, and on page 3, Part IV, line 6.

Column 3--Divide the allocated expense in column 1 by the
inpatient days in column 2 to arrive at the average per diem cost.

Column 4--Enter in column 4, the title XVIII - Part B inpatient
days for each patient care area. These days are obtained from
page 2, Part II, line 10k, or from page 3, Part IV, line 10k, as
appropriate.

Column 5--Multiply the average per diem cost in column 3 by the
number of inpatient days in column 4 to arrive at the expense
applicable to title XVIII.

The expenses entered on lines 7, 8, 9 and 10 should be
transferred to the appropriate lines on Part III, column 4,
whenever both Parts I and II are completed.

However, when only Part II is completed, the expenses entered on
lines 7, 8, 9 and 10 should be transferred directly to Worksheet E,
Part I, columns 2, 4, 6 and 8, as appropriate, line 4.

336.3 Part III - Summary for Title XVIII (To be completed only if
both Parts I and II are used).--This part is applicable to
Medicare only and is provided to summarize the amounts apportioned
to the program in Parts I and II. This part is completed only if
both Parts I and II are used.

338.   WORKSHEET D-3 - APPORTIONMENT OF HOSPITAL-BASED PHYSICIAN
       REMUNERATION FOR PROFESSIONAL SERVICES - COMBINED BILLING
This worksheet is provided to apportion to titles V, XVIII and
XIX the remuneration for professional services rendered by
hospital-based physicians using combined billing. A separate
copy of this worksheet must be completed for the hospital and
each subprovider.

This worksheet provides for all hospital departments under which
combined billing may be used. (See the Hospital Manual (HIM-10),
chapter 4.) With respect to the departments listed on this worksheet, if separate billing and cost data are not maintained for
radiology-diagnostic, radiology-therapeutic and radioisotope,
enter the total radiology department data on line 1 (Radiology -
Diagnostic).

Column 1--Enter in column 1 on the appropriate lines, the total
remuneration for professional services applicable to each
hospital department under which combined billing is used. These
amounts must be obtained from the provider's records and should
agree with the amounts entered on Worksheet A-8 relative to
adjustments eliminating the total remuneration for professional
services from allowable cost.

Column 2--Enter on the appropriate line in this column, the
total charges (inpatient and outpatient) to all patients for each
department.

NOTE: If the provider has elected to be reimbursed for kidney
       acquisition costs under the ALTERNATIVE PROCEDURES as
       explained in the instructions to Supplemental Worksheet D-6,
       the kidney acquisition charges should be eliminated from
       the total charges in this column.

Column 3--Divide the remuneration in column 1 for each department
under which combined billing is used by the total charges in
column 2 and enter the resulting ratios in column 3.

Columns 4a through 4e--Enter in the appropriate columns that
portion of the total charges in column 2 which is applicable to
title V (inpatient), title XVIII (inpatient), title XVIII -
Part B (outpatient), title XIX (inpatient) and kidney acquisition
(inpatient and outpatient), respectively. The inpatient charges
applicable to title XVIII include those billed on form HCFA-1453
as well as those inpatient charges billed on form HCFA-1483
(inpatient billing form when Part A benefits are not available).

No entry should be made in column 4e if the provider has elected
to be reimbursed for kidney acquisition costs under the ALTERNA-
TIVE PROCEDURES as explained in the instructions to Supplemental
Worksheet D-6.

NOTE: If gross combined charges for professional and provider
       component are used on Worksheet C, gross combined charges
       must be used on this worksheet. If gross charges for
       provider component only are used on Worksheet C, gross
       charges for professional component only must be used on
       this worksheet.

       Likewise, if gross combined charges, for professional and
       provider component are used in column 2, then combined charges
       must be used in columns 4a through 4e. If gross charges for
       professional component only are used in column 2, then gross
       charges for professional component only must be used in
       columns 4a through 4e.

Columns 5a through 5e--For each medical specialty department,
multiply the ratio of total remuneration to total charges in
column 3 by the health care program charges in columns 4a, 4b, 4c,
4d and 4e, respectively. Enter the resulting amounts in columns
5a, 5b, 5c, 5d and 5e, as appropriate.

339. WORKSHEET D-8 - APPORTIONMENT OF MALPRACTICE INSURANCE COSTS
The purpose of this worksheet is to compute the amount of malpractice
insurance premiums or malpractice insurance fund contributions
that is to be included as a title V, title XVIII and title XIX
reimbursable cost.

NOTE: Where the amount of malpractice insurance premiums and/or
       fund contributions applicable to each component of the
       health care complex can be specifically identified, a
       separate copy of this worksheet must be completed for each
       component. In this situation, the lines applicable to the
       home health agency are not completed. For other health
       care complex components, lines 10 and 11 are not completed
       but all other lines for such components are completed.

If a provider pays allowable uninsured malpractice losses incurred
by health care program patients, either through allowable deductible
or coinsurance provisions or as a result of an award in excess of
reasonable coverage limits, or as a governmental provider, such
losses and related direct costs are directly assigned to the
appropriate health care program in Part III and Part IV.

339.1 Part I - Paid Malpractice Losses.--

Lines 1 through 6--Enter on these lines in the appropriate columns
the amount of malpractice losses paid by and on behalf of the
provider, excluding those amounts applicable to the hospital-based
home health agency. Do not enter any amounts for contingent losses,
that is, pending claims or claims that are in dispute.

Rev. 10   3-63

339.2 Part II - Apportionment to Health Care Programs.--

Line 7--This line only needs to be completed when there are no
entries on lines 1 through 6. Enter for each health care program,
the national ratio of malpractice awards paid to health care
patients to malpractice awards paid to all patients. The title XIX
ratio will be used for title V until a separate title V ratio is
developed (title XVIII 5.1%; title XIX 7.5%).

Lines 8 through 10--The ratios entered on these lines must be
rounded to eight decimal places.

Line 11--Enter the amount of malpractice insurance premiums or
fund contributions. This amount is the malpractice insurance
premiums and/or fund contributions from Worksheet A-8, column 2,
line 35.

Line 12--This line is necessary to compute the amount of
malpractice insurance premiums and/or fund contributions applicable
to the home health agency. The ratio on this line must be rounded
to eight decimal places.

339.3 Part III - Directly Assigned Malpractice Costs - Title V
and Title XIX.--

Lines 20 through 22--Enter on these lines the amount from
Worksheet A-8 for paid malpractice losses and related direct
expenses for title V and for title XIX. Use the ratios in column 2,
lines 17a through 17c (title V) or lines 19a through 19c (title XIX)
in determining the amount applicable to hospital, subprovider I
and subprovider II. The total of these lines must equal the amounts
on Worksheet A-8, column 2, lines 38 and 39, for title XIX and
lines 40 and 41 for title V.

Transfer the sum of lines 17 or 19 and 20, 21 or 22 for each
component to Worksheet E-5, Part I, line 5, column as appropriate.

339.4 Part IV - Directly Assigned Malpractice Costs - Title XVIII.--

Lines 23 through 26--Enter on these lines the adjustment from
Worksheet A-8 for paid malpractice losses and related direct
expenses for title XVIII. Use the ratios in column 2, lines 18a
through 18h in determining the amount applicable to the hospital,
skilled nursing facility and each component. The total of these
lines must equal the amounts on Worksheet A-8, column 2, lines 36
and 37.

Transfer the costs on lines 18a through 18h, column 3, plus the
amounts for the corresponding component cost on lines 23 through
26, columns 1 and 2, to Worksheet E, Part I, line 10, column as
appropriate.

340. WORKSHEET E - CALCULATION OF REIMBURSEMENT SETTLEMENT -
      TITLE XVIII - PART A AND PART B SERVICES
This worksheet applies to title XVIII only and provides for the
reimbursement calculation of Part A and Part B services rendered
to Medicare patients by the provider and provider components of
the health care complex.

Worksheet E consists of the following three parts:

>   Part I   - Computation of Net Cost of Medicare Covered
>   Services
>   Part II   - Computation of the Lesser of Reasonable Cost
>   or Customary Charges
>   Part III - Computation of Reimbursement Settlement

340.1 Part I - Computation of Net Cost of Medicare Covered
Services.--

LINE DESCRIPTIONS

Lines 1 through 11--Enter in the appropriate column on lines 1
through 10, the indicated costs for each component of the health
care complex.

The amount to be entered on line 2 is the title XVIII, Part B,
outpatient service costs from Worksheet C, column 7, as follows:

>   a. Target Rate Reimbursement Elected - From Worksheet C,
> column 7, line 34a minus line 29a.

>   b. Cost Reimbursement - From Worksheet C, column 7,
> line 34a.

The amount to be entered on line 5 is the Medicare program's
share of the reasonable compensation paid to physicians for
services on utilization review committees applicable to the
skilled nursing facility. The amount on this line should have
been included in the amount eliminated from total costs on
Worksheet A-8, line 58.

Enter on line 9, the cost of services furnished "under arrangements"
to Medicare beneficiaries only (see PRM, Part I, chapter 21).

Enter on line 11, the sum of the amounts on lines 1 through 10.

Line 12--Enter in the appropriate columns 1, 3, 5 and 7, the
applicable charge differential between semiprivate and less than
semiprivate accommodations. The amount of the differential is the
difference between the provider's customary charge for semiprivate accommodations and its customary charge for the less than
semiprivate accommodations furnished for all Medicare patient

days where the accommodations furnished were provided not at the patients' request, nor for a reason which is consistent with program purposes.

Line 13--Enter the total amount of kidney acquisition charges billed to Medicare under Part B on form HCFA-1483. This would occur when kidneys are transplanted into Medicare beneficiaries who on the day of transplantation are not entitled to or have exhausted Part A benefits. This computation reflects an adjustment between Medicare Part A and Part B costs so that the amount added under Part B is the same amount to be subtracted under Part A for the appropriate hospital or subprovider.

Line 15--Enter any amounts paid and payable by workers' compensation. Such amounts should be for the cost of services which is included in the Medicare program's share of allowable costs. Generally, such amounts are applicable to routine services.

Line 16--Enter the total revenue applicable to kidneys furnished to other providers, kidney procurement organizations and others and for kidneys transplanted into non-Medicare patients. Such revenues must be determined under the accrual method of accounting. If kidneys are transplanted into non-Medicare patients who are not liable for payment on a charge basis, and as such, there is no revenue applicable to the related kidney acquisitions, the amount entered on line 16 must also include an amount representing the acquisition cost of the kidneys transplanted into such patients. This amount should be determined by multiplying the average cost of kidney acquisition by the number of kidneys transplanted into non-Medicare patients who are not liable for payment on a charge basis. The average cost of kidney acquisition is computed by dividing the total cost of kidney acquisition (including the inpatient routine service costs and the inpatient ancillary service costs applicable to kidney acquisition, which have been included in Medicare costs) by the total number of kidneys transplanted into all patients and furnished to others. If the average cost cannot be determined in the manner described, then the appropriate standard kidney acquisition charge should be used in lieu of the average cost.

Lines 17 and 22--Enter in the appropriate columns on these lines, the professional remuneration paid to hospital-based physicians for services rendered to Medicare beneficiaries. These lines will be completed only when combined billing is used.

340.2 Part II - Computation of the Lesser of Reasonable Cost or Customary Charges.--Providers will be paid the lesser of the reasonable cost of services furnished to beneficiaries or the customary charges made by the provider for the same services. This part provides for the computation of the lesser of

reasonable cost as defined in Health Insurance Regulations
section 405.455(b)(2) or customary charges as defined in Health
Insurance Regulations section 405.455(b)(1).

LINE DESCRIPTIONS

Lines 1 through 5--These lines provide for the computation of
reasonable cost of title XVIII - Part A and Part B services.

Lines 6 through 15--These lines provide for the accumulation of
charges which relate to the reasonable cost on line 5.

Do not include on these lines (1) the portion of charges applicable
to the excess costs of luxury items or services (see PRM,
Part I, chapter 21), (2) provider charges to beneficiaries for
excess costs as described in PRM, Part I, chapter 25, and (3) the
standard kidney acquisition charges billed to the program for
kidneys transplanted into Medicare beneficiaries.

With respect to (3) above, in lieu of the standard kidney
acquisition charges, the detailed departmental charges generated in
the course of kidney acquisitions and which may be reflected as
"memoranda billings" should be included in the customary charges
reflected on lines 7, 9 and 12, as appropriate.

The adjustment between Part A and Part B charges for the total
amount of kidney acquisition charges billed to Medicare under
Part B on form HCFA-1483 will be shown on line 14. This would
occur when kidneys are transplanted into Medicare beneficiaries
who on the day of transplantation are not entitled to or have
exhausted Part A benefits. This computation reflects an adjustment between Medicare Part A and Part B charges so that the amount
added under Part B is the same amount to be subtracted under
Part A for the appropriate hospital or subprovider.

Enter on lines 7 and 8, the Medicare charges for inpatient
ancillary and for outpatient services, respectively. If the
charges on Worksheets C and D do not include the professional
component of hospital-based physician remuneration, the amounts
to be entered on line 7 should be obtained from the appropriate
Worksheet D, columns 3 and 4, line 28, and the amount to be
entered on line 8 should be obtained from Worksheet C, column 7,
line 34b. However, if the provider elected the target rate
reimbursement for home program dialysis, exclude the charges from
Worksheet C, column 7, line 29b.

If the charges on Worksheets C and D do include such professional
component, the amount of the professional component should be
eliminated from the charges to be entered on lines 7 and 8.

The amounts entered on line 9 should include covered late charges
which have been billed to the program where the patient's medical
condition is the cause of the stay past the check-out time. Also,
these amounts should include charges relating to a stay in a
special care unit for a few hours where the provider's normal
practice is to bill for the partial stay. In addition, these
charges should include the charges for semiprivate accommodations
of Medicare inpatients for which workers' compensation was paid
at the ward rate and will subsequently be deducted from final
settlement.

The amounts entered on line 13 are for services furnished
"under arrangements" to Medicare beneficiaries only. (See PRM,
Part I, chapter 21.)

Lines 16 through 20--These lines provide for the reduction of
Medicare charges where the provider does not actually impose such
charges in the case of most patients liable for payment for
services on a charge basis or fails to make reasonable efforts to
collect such charges from those patients. Providers which do
impose these charges and make reasonable efforts to collect the
charges from patients liable for payment for services on a charge
basis are not required to complete lines 17 through 19, but should
enter on line 20 the amount from line 15. See Health Insurance
Regulations 405.455(b). In no instance may the customary charges
on line 20 exceed the actual charge on line 15.

340.3   Part III - Computation of Reimbursement Settlement.--

LINE DESCRIPTIONS

Line 14--Enter on this line the program's share of any net
depreciation adjustment applicable to prior years resulting from
the gain or loss on the disposition of depreciable assets. (See
PRM, Part I, chapter 1.) Enter the amount of any excess
depreciation taken in parenthesis (   ).

Line 15--Enter on this line the program's share of any recovery
of excess depreciation applicable to prior years resulting from
provider termination or a decrease in Medicare utilization. (See
PRM, Part I, chapter 1.)

Line 16--Where a provider's cost limit is raised as a result of
its request for review, amounts which were erroneously collected
on the basis of the initial cost limit are required to be
refunded to the beneficiary. Enter on this line any amounts
which are not refunded, either because they are less than $5
collected from a beneficiary or because the provider is unable
to locate the beneficiary. (See PRM, Part I, chapter 25.)

342. WORKSHEET E-1 - ANALYSIS OF PAYMENTS TO PROVIDERS FOR
      SERVICES RENDERED TO TITLE XVIII (MEDICARE) BENEFICIARIES
This worksheet must be completed for each component of the health
care complex which has a separate provider or subprovider number
as shown on page 1, item I. This worksheet should be completed for
only Medicare interim payments. It should <u>not</u> be completed for
purposes of reporting interim payments for titles V and XIX, for
delegated PSRO review and for home program dialysis payments
under the target rate reimbursement option. The column headings
designate three categories of payments:

        Category 1 - Inpatient Part A
        Category 2 - Inpatient Part B
        Category 3 - Outpatient Part B

Providers should complete lines 1 through 4. <u>The remainder of
the worksheet will be completed by your intermediary.</u> All amounts
to be reported on this worksheet must be for services, the cost of
which is included in this cost report.

<u>NOTE</u>: When completing the heading, enter the provider number
      which corresponds to the provider, subprovider or skilled
      nursing facility which is checked off.

<u>Line 1</u>--Enter on this line the total Medicare interim payments
paid to the provider (excluding PSRO review payments and home
program dialysis - other payments where the target rate election
is made). The amount entered must reflect the sum of all interim
payments paid on individual bills (net of adjustment bills) for
services rendered in this cost reporting period. The amount
entered on this line must include amounts withheld from the
provider's interim payments due to a set off against overpayments
to the provider applicable to to prior cost reporting periods.
Also, include the total Medicare payments for home program renal
dialysis equipment where the provider elected 100 percent cost
reimbursement. It should not include any retroactive lump sum
adjustment amounts based on a subsequent revision of the interim
rate, or tentative or net settlement amounts; nor should it include
interim payments payable. If the provider is reimbursed under the
periodic interim payment method of reimbursement, enter on this
line the periodic interim payments received for this cost reporting period.

<u>Line 2</u>--Enter on this line the total Medicare interim payments
(excluding PSRO review payments and home program dialysis other
payments where the target rate reimbursement election is made)
payable on individual bills. Since the cost in the cost report
is on an accrual basis, this line represents the amount of
services rendered in the cost reporting period, but not paid as
of the end of the cost reporting period.

Also, include on this line the total Medicare payments payable for home program renal dialysis equipment where the provider elected 100 percent cost reimbursement.

Line 3--Enter on this line the amount of each retroactive lump sum adjustment and the applicable date.

Line 4--Enter on this line the total amount of the interim payments (sum of lines 1, 2 and 3k). Transfer these totals to the appropriate column on Worksheet E, Part III, line 18.

PROVIDERS DO NOT COMPLETE THE REMAINDER OF WORKSHEET E-1. THE REMAINDER OF THE WORKSHEET WILL BE COMPLETED BY YOUR INTERMEDIARY.

344.   WORKSHEET E-2 - CALCULATION OF REIMBURSABLE BAD DEBTS -
       TITLE XVIII - PART B
This worksheet provides for the calculation of reimbursable Medicare Part B bad debts. Bad debts for deductible and coinsurance amounts attributable to the professional component services of hospital-based physicians are not reimbursable under the Medicare program. If hospitals using combined billing do not identify bad debts related to physician professional services and to provider services, or analyze the records to separately identify these, such hospitals must calculate and eliminate the professional component bad debts from the total Part B bad debts. Column 1, lines 13, 14 and 15 provide for this optional calculation. (See PRM, Part I, chapter 3.)

Line 1--When professional component bad debts are eliminated from Part B debts, the amounts on this line are determined as follows: For columns 1 or 4, from Worksheet E, Part I, columns 2 or 8, as appropriate, line 14 minus Worksheet E, Part II, columns 2 or 8, as appropriate, line 4; for columns 2 or 3, from Worksheet E, Part I, columns 4 or 6, as appropriate, line 14.

When professional component bad debts are not eliminated from Part B debts, the amounts on this line are determined as follows: For columns 1 or 4, from Worksheet E, Part I, columns 2 or 8, as appropriate, line 18 minus Worksheet E, Part II, columns 2 or 8, as appropriate, line 4; for columns 2 or 3, from Worksheet E, Part I, columns 4 or 6, as appropriate, line 18. Column 1, lines 13, 14 and 15 must be completed for computing the professional component bad debts included in the bad debts.

Line 2--The amounts to be entered on this line are determined as follows: For columns 1 and 4, hospitals and skilled nursing facilities which are not hospital based, multiply the amount on line 1, columns 1 or 4 times the ratio from Supplemental Worksheet F, Part III, line 3. For columns 2 through 4, subproviders

and hospital-based skilled nursing facilities, obtain the amount
from Worksheet E, Part II, columns 4, 6 and 8, line 3.

Line 4--When professional component bad debts are eliminated from
Part B bad debts, the amounts on this line are determined as
follows: For columns 1 or 4, from Worksheet E, Part I, columns 2
or 8, line 14 minus line 19 times 80 percent, plus Worksheet E,
Part III, columns 2 or 8, line 2 minus Worksheet E, Part III,
columns 2 or 8, line 3; for columns 2 or 3, from Worksheet E,
Part I, columns 4 or 6, line 21 plus Worksheet E, Part III,
columns 4 or 6, line 2.

When professional component bad debts are not eliminated from
Part B bad debts, the amounts on this line are determined as
follows: For columns 1 or 4, from Worksheet E, Part I,
columns 2 or 8, line 21 plus Worksheet E, Part III, columns 2
or 8, line 2 minus Worksheet E, Part III, columns 2 or 8,
line 3; for columns 2 or 3, from Worksheet E, Part I, columns 4
or 6, line 21 plus Worksheet E, Part III, columns 4 or 6,
line 21 plus Worksheet E, Part III, columns 4 or 6, line 2.

Lines 6, 7 and 8--When professional component bad debts are
eliminated from Part B bad debts, lines 6, 7 and 8 must not
include any charges for physician professional services.

Lines 11 and 13 through 15--Column 1 for these lines must be
completed for computing the professional component bad debts
included in the bad debts.

346. WORKSHEET E-5 - CALCULATION OF REIMBURSEMENT SETTLEMENT
This worksheet provides for the reimbursement calculation of the
cost of services rendered to title V and title XIX health care
program inpatients by the provider and subproviders of the health
care complex. A separate copy of this worksheet should be
completed for title V and for title XIX.

Worksheet E-5 consists of the following three parts:

       Part I   - Computation of Net Cost of Covered Services
       Part II   - Computation of Lesser of Reasonable Cost or
                     Customary Charges
       Part III - Computation of Reimbursement Settlement

346.1 Part I - Computation of Net Cost of Covered Services.--

LINE DESCRIPTIONS

Lines 1 through 7--Enter in the appropriate column on lines 1 through
6, the indicated costs for each component of the health care complex.

If appropriate, enter on line 6, the kidney acquisition costs applicable to patients covered under title V or title XIX, but who are not covered under title XVIII. The costs should be determined in the manner described in the instructions for Worksheet E, Part I, line 16.

Line 8--Enter in the appropriate column the applicable charge differential between semiprivate and less than semiprivate accommodations. The amount of the differential is the difference between the provider's customary charge for the less than semiprivate accommodations and its customary charge for the accommodations furnished for all health care program patient days where the accommodations furnished were provided not at the patient's request, nor for a reason which is consistent with health care program purposes.

Line 10--Enter in the appropriate columns the professional remuneration paid to hospital-based physicians for inpatient services rendered to health care program beneficiaries. These lines will be completed only when combined billing is used.

Line 11--Enter any amounts paid and payable by workers' compensation. Such amounts should be for the cost of services which is included in the health care program's share of allowable costs. Generally, such amounts are applicable to routine services.

346.2   Part II - Computation of the Lesser of Reasonable Cost or Customary Charges.--Providers will be paid the lesser of the reasonable cost of services furnished to beneficiaries or the customary charges made by the provider for the same services. This part provides for the computation of the lesser of reasonable cost as defined in Health Insurance Regulations section 405.455 (b)(2) or customary charges as defined in Health Insurance Regulations section 405.455(b)(1).

LINE DESCRIPTIONS

Lines 1 through 4--These lines provide for the computation of reasonable cost of inpatient services applicable to the health care program.

Lines 5 through 10--These lines provide for the accumulation of charges which relate to the reasonable cost on line 4.

Do not include on these lines the portion of charges applicable to the excess costs of luxury items or services (see PRM, Part I, chapter 21).

Enter on line 6, the health care program charges for inpatient ancillary services. If the charges on Worksheet D do not include the professional component of   hospital-based physician

Exhibit 18

FORM APPROVED
OMB NO. 0938-0050

COMPUTATION OF INPATIENT ROUTINE SERVICE COST

PROVIDER NO.		PERIOD FROM ___ TO ___	WORKSHEET D-1 PART I

PART 1 — TITLE XVIII (MEDICARE)

GENERAL INPATIENT CARE UNITS (EXCLUDING NURSERY) COST

INPATIENT DAYS

		Hospital 1	Subprovider 2	Subprovider 3	Skilled Nursing Facility 4	
1	Total aged, pediatric and maternity inpatient days (Fr page 3, Pt II, col 1, line 4, page 4, Pt IV, col. as applicable, line 4)					1
2	Total other than aged, pediatric and maternity inpatient days (excl. newborn) (Fr pg 3, Pt II, col 1, line 5, pg 4, Pt IV, col as appl. line 5)					2
3	Total inpatient days—all patients (excl. newborn) (Sum of lines 1 & 2; must agree with pg 3, Pt II, col 1, line 6; pg 4, Pt IV, cols as appl. line 6)					3
4	Aged, pediatric and maternity inpatient days plus inpatient routine nursing salary cost differential (SEE INSTRUCTIONS)					4
5	Total adjusted inpatient days (Sum of lines 2 and 4)					5
6	Aged, pediatric and maternity inpatient days—appl. to title XVIII, Pt A (Fr pg 3, Pt II, col 1, line 10c; pg 4, Pt IV, col. as appl., line 10)					6
7	Other than aged, pediatric & maternity inpatient days—appl. to title XVIII, Pt A (Fr pg 3, Pt II, col 1, line 10f; pg 4, Pt IV, col as appl., line 10f)					7
8	Total inpatient days appl. to title XVIII, Pt A (Sum of lines 6&7; must agree with pg 3, Pt II, col 1, line 10f; pg 4, Pt IV, col as appl., line 10f)					8
	INPATIENT ROUTINE COSTS					
9	Total inpatient routine nursing salary cost (excluding nursery)	$	$	$	$	9
10	Total inpatient routine service cost (excluding inpatient routine nursing salary cost on line 9)					10
11	Total inpatient routine service cost (Sum of lines 9 and 10)	$	$	$	$	11
12	Inpatient routine nursing salary cost plus inpatient routine nursing salary cost differential (SEE INSTRUCTIONS)	$	$	$	$	12
	MEDICARE GENERAL INPATIENT CARE PER DIEM COSTS (including the Inpatient Routine Nursing Salary Cost Differential Adjustment Factor)					
13	Adjusted avg per diem inpatient routine nursing salary cost appl. to aged, pediatric & maternity patients incl. the inpatient routine nursing salary cost differential adjustment factor (line 12 ÷ line 5)	$	$	$	$	13
14	Average per diem inpatient routine nursing salary cost (excl. inpatient routine nursing salary cost) (Line 10 ÷ line 3)					14
15	Adjusted avg per diem inpatient routine service cost appl. to aged, pediatric & maternity patients including the inpatient routine nursing salary cost differential adjustment factor (Sum of lines 13 and 14)	$	$	$	$	15
16	Total inpatient routine service cost (line 11)	$	$	$	$	16
17	Inpatient routine service cost appl. to all aged, pediatric & maternity patients (line 1 × line 15)					17
18	Inpatient routine service cost appl. to all patients—other than aged, pediatric & maternity (line 16 minus line 17)	$	$	$	$	18
19	Avg per diem inpatient routine service cost appl. to all patients—other than aged, pediatric & maternity (line 18 ÷ line 2)	$	$	$	$	19
	MEDICARE GENERAL INPATIENT ROUTINE SERVICE COST BEFORE ROUTINE SERVICE COST LIMITATION					
20	Medicare general inpatient routine service cost appl. to aged, pediatric & maternity patients (line 6 × line 15)	$	$	$	$	20
21	Medicare general inpatient routine service cost appl. to all patients—other than aged, pediatric & maternity (line 7 × line 19)					21
22	Total Medicare general inpatient routine service cost before reasonable cost limitation (Sum of lines 20 and 21)	$	$	$	$	22
23	Aggregate charges to beneficiaries for excess costs (From provider records) (SEE INSTRUCTIONS)	( )	( )	( )	( )	23
24	TOTAL (Line 22 minus line 23)	$	$	$	$	24

FORM HCFA-2552-81 (11-81)

24

Exhibit 18 continued

FORM APPROVED
OMB NO. 0938-0050

COMPUTATION OF INPATIENT ROUTINE SERVICE COST	WORKSHEET D-1 PART 1

PROVIDER NO.:	PERIOD: FROM _____ TO _____

PART I—TITLE XVIII (MEDICARE)

25 Allocation of capital related costs to general inpatient routine service cost centers for general inpatient routine service cost limitation application

		Directly Assigned Capital Related Costs	DEPRECIATION BUILDINGS & FIXTURES	DEPRECIATION MOVABLE EQUIPMENT	DEPRECIATION TO BE ALLOCATED (Sum of cols 0-2)	EMPLOYEE HEALTH & WELFARE	
		0	1	2	3	4	
.4	Employee Health & Welfare	$	$	$	$	$	.4
.5	Administrative & General						.5
.6	Maintenance & Repairs						.6
.7	Operation of Plant						.7
.8	Laundry & Linen Service						.8
.9	Housekeeping						.9
.10	Dietary						.10
.11	Cafeteria						.11
.12	Maintenance of Personnel						.12
.13	Nursing Administration						.13
.14	Central Services & Supply						.14
.15	Pharmacy						.15
.16	Medical Records & Library						.16
.17	Social Services						.17
.18	Nursing School						.18
.19	Intern-Resident Service (in approved teach. prog.)						.19
.20							.20
.46	Adults & Pediatrics (General Routine Care)						.46
.49							.49
.50							.50
.52	Skilled Nursing Facility-Certified						.52
AA	Sum of other cost centers (SEE INSTRUCTIONS)						AA
AB	Adjustment (SEE INSTRUCTIONS)						AB
BB	TOTAL (Sum of lines 25.4 to 25.AB)	$	$	$	$	$	BB

26 Statistics used in the allocation of capital related costs to general inpatient routine service cost centers

		EMPLOYEE HEALTH & WELFARE	
		4	
.4	Employee Health & Welfare	$	.4
.5	Administrative & General		.5
.6	Maintenance & Repairs		.6
.7	Operation of Plant		.7
.8	Laundry & Linen Service		.8
.9	Housekeeping		.9
.10	Dietary		.10
.11	Cafeteria		.11
.12	Maintenance of Personnel		.12
.13	Nursing Administration		.13
.14	Central Services & Supply		.14
.15	Pharmacy		.15
.16	Medical Records & Library		.16
.17	Social Services		.17
.18	Nursing School		.18
.19	Intern-Resident Service (in approved teach. prog.)		.19
.20			.20
.46	Adults & Pediatrics (General Routine Care)		.46
.49			.49
.50			.50
.52	Skilled Nursing Facility-Certified		.52
AA	Sum of other cost centers (SEE INSTRUCTIONS)		AA
27	Cost to be Allocated	$	27
28	Unit Cost Multiplier		28

Exhibit 18 continued

COMPUTATION OF INPATIENT ROUTINE SERVICE COST	WORKSHEET D-1 PART 1 Continued

PROVIDER NO.:	PERIOD: FROM _____ TO _____

PART I—TITLE XVIII (MEDICARE)

25

	ADMINISTRATIVE & GENERAL	MAINTENANCE & REPAIRS	OPERATION OF PLANT	LAUNDRY & LINEN SERVICE	HOUSEKEEPING	DIETARY	CAFETERIA	
	5	6	7	8	9	10	11	
.4	▨							.4
.5	$							.5
.6		$						.6
.7			$					.7
.8				$				.8
.9					$			.9
.10						$		.10
.11							$	.11
.12								.12
.13								.13
.14								.14
.15								.15
.16								.16
.17								.17
.18								.18
.19								.19
.20								.20
.46								.46
.49								.49
.50								.50
.52								.52
.AA								.AA
.AB								.AB
.BB	$	$	$	$	$	$	$	.BB

26

	ADMINISTRATIVE & GENERAL	MAINTENANCE & REPAIRS	OPERATION OF PLANT	LAUNDRY & LINEN SERVICE	HOUSEKEEPING	DIETARY	CAFETERIA	
	5	6	7	8	9	10	11	
.4	▨							.4
.5	$							.5
.6								.6
.7								.7
.8								.8
.9								.9
.10								.10
.11								.11
.12								.12
.13								.13
.14								.14
.15								.15
.16								.16
.17								.17
.18								.18
.19								.19
.20								.20
.46								.46
.49								.49
.50								.50
.52								.52
.AA								.AA
27	$	$	$	$	$	$	$	27
28								28

Exhibit 18 continued

FORM APPROVED
OMB NO. 0938-0060

COMPUTATION OF INPATIENT ROUTINE SERVICE COST	WORKSHEET D-1 PART 1

PROVIDER NO.: _____

PERIOD:
FROM _____
TO _____

PART I—TITLE XVIII (MEDICARE)

25 Allocation of capital related costs to general inpatient routine service cost centers
    for general inpatient routine service cost limitation application

		MAINTENANCE OF PERSONNEL	NURSING ADMINISTRATION	CENTRAL SERVICES & SUPPLY	
		12	13	14	
.4	Employee Health & Welfare				.4
.5	Administrative & General				.5
.6	Maintenance & Repairs				.6
.7	Operation of Plant				.7
.8	Laundry & Linen Service				.8
.9	Housekeeping				.9
.10	Dietary				.10
.11	Cafeteria				.11
.12	Maintenance of Personnel	$			.12
.13	Nursing Administration		$		.13
.14	Central Services & Supply			$	.14
.15	Pharmacy				.15
.16	Medical Records & Library				.16
.17	Social Services				.17
.18	Nursing School				.18
.19	Intern-Resident Service (in approved teach. prog.)				.19
.20					.20
.46	Adults & Pediatrics (General Routine Care)				.46
.49					.49
.50					.50
.52	Skilled Nursing Facility-Certified				.52
.AA	Sum of other cost centers (SEE INSTRUCTIONS)				.AA
.AB	Adjustment (SEE INSTRUCTIONS)				.AB
BB	TOTAL (Sum of lines 25.4 to 25.AB)	$	$	$	BB

26 Statistics used in the allocation of capital related costs to general inpatient routine
    service cost centers

		MAINTENANCE OF PERSONNEL	NURSING ADMINISTRATION	CENTRAL SERVICES & SUPPLY	
		12	13	14	
.4	Employee Health & Welfare				.4
.5	Administrative & General				.5
.6	Maintenance & Repairs				.6
.7	Operation of Plant				.7
.8	Laundry & Linen Service				.8
.9	Housekeeping				.9
.10	Dietary				.10
.11	Cafeteria				.11
.12	Maintenance of Personnel				.12
.13	Nursing Administration				.13
.14	Central Services & Supply			$	.14
.15	Pharmacy				.15
.16	Medical Records & Library				.16
.17	Social Services				.17
.18	Nursing School				.18
.19	Intern-Resident Service (in approved teach. prog.)				.19
.20					.20
.46	Adults & Pediatrics (General Routine Care)				.46
.49					.49
.50					.50
.52	Skilled Nursing Facility-Certified				.52
.AA	Sum of other cost centers (SEE INSTRUCTIONS)				.AA
27	Cost to be Allocated	$	$	$	27
28	Unit Cost Multiplier				28

FORM HCFA-2552-81 (11-81)

26

Exhibit 18 continued

COMPUTATION OF INPATIENT ROUTINE SERVICE COST	WORKSHEET D-1 PART 1 Continued

	PROVIDER NO.:	PERIOD: FROM _____ TO _____

PART I—TITLE XVIII (MEDICARE)

25

	PHARMACY	MEDICAL RECORDS & LIBRARY	SOCIAL SERVICES	NURSING SCHOOL	INTERN-RESIDENT SERVICE (in approved teaching program)		TOTAL (Sum of cols 3-20)	
	15	16	17	18	19	20	21	
.4								.4
.5								.5
.6								.6
.7								.7
.8								.8
.9								.9
.10								.10
.11								.11
.12								.12
.13								.13
.14								.14
.15	$							.15
.16		$						.16
.17			$					.17
.18				$				.18
.19					$			.19
.20						$		.20
.46							$	.46
.49							$	.49
.50							$	.50
.52							$	.52
AA							$	AA
AB							$	AB
BB	$	$	$	$	$	$	$	BB

26

	PHARMACY	MEDICAL RECORDS & LIBRARY	SOCIAL SERVICES	NURSING SCHOOL	INTERN-RESIDENT SERVICE (in approved teaching program)			
	15	16	17	18	19	20	21	
.4								.4
.5								.5
.6								.6
.7								.7
.8								.8
.9								.9
.10								.10
.11								.11
.12								.12
.13								.13
.14								.14
.15	$							.15
.16								.16
.17								.17
.18								.18
.19								.19
.20								.20
.46								.46
.49								.49
.50								.50
.52								.52
AA								AA
27	$	$	$	$	$	$		27
28								28

26 continued

FORM HCFA-2552-81 (11-81)

Exhibit 18 continued

FORM APPROVED
OMB NO. 0938-0050

WORKSHEET D-1

COMPUTATION OF INPATIENT ROUTINE SERVICE COST

PROVIDER NO. _____   PERIOD FROM _____ TO _____

PART I — TITLE XVIII (Medicare)

MEDICARE GENERAL INPATIENT ROUTINE SERVICE COST

	HOSPITAL 1	SUBPROVIDER -1 2	SUBPROVIDER -II 3	SKILLED NURSING FACILITY 4
29 Depreciation allocated to general inpatient routine service (From column 21, line 25.46 [hospital]; line 25.49 and/or line 25.50 [subprovider]; line 25.52 [skilled nursing facility])	$	$	$	$
30 Cost of approved medical education programs (From Wkst. B, sum of columns 18 and 19, line 46 [hospital], lines 49 and/or 50 [subprovider])				
31 Total cost to be excluded from general inpatient routine service cost (sum of lines 29 and 30)	$	$	$	$
32 Per diem for excludable cost (line 31 ÷ line 3)	$	$	$	$
33 Medicare excludable cost (line 32 × line 8)	$	$	$	$
34 General inpatient routine service cost for comparison to cost limitation (line 24 minus line 33)	$	$	$	$
35 General inpatient routine service cost limitation (line 8 × $ _____ per diem limitation [hospital/subprovider]; line 8 × $ _____ per diem limitation [skilled nursing facility])	$	$	$	$
36 Aggregate charges for excess cost applicable to kidney acquisition (From page 3, Part II, line 10h or page 4, Part IV, line 10h × $ _____ per diem charge)	$	$	$	$
37 TOTAL (Sum of lines 35 and 36)	$	$	$	$
38 Reimbursable general inpatient routine service cost (if line 34 is less than line 37, enter the sum of lines 33 and 34) (if line 37 is less than line 34, enter the sum of lines 33 and 37)	$	$	$	$

INTENSIVE CARE TYPE INPATIENT HOSPITAL UNITS

INTENSIVE CARE TYPE INPATIENT HOSPITAL UNITS	TOTAL INPATIENT COST 1	TOTAL INPATIENT DAYS 2	AVERAGE PER DIEM (COL. 1 ÷ COL. 2) 3	MEDICARE DAYS 4	COST APPLIC. TO MEDICARE (COL. 3 × COL. 4) 5
39 Intensive Care Unit	$		$		$
40 Coronary Care Unit	$		$		$
41	$		$		$
42	$		$		$
43 TOTAL MEDICARE INPATIENT GENERAL ROUTINE AND INTENSIVE CARE TYPE INPATIENT HOSPITAL (Sum of lines 38—42) (Transfer to Worksheet E, Part 1, column as appropriate, line 3)					$

FORM HCFA-2552-81 (11-81)

27

Exhibit 19

FORM APPROVED
OMB NO. 0938-0050

WORKSHEET D-1
PART II

COMPUTATION OF INPATIENT ROUTINE SERVICE COST

PROVIDER NO. ___ PERIOD: FROM ___ TO ___

CHECK ONE: ☐ TITLE V ☐ TITLE XIX

	HOSPITAL 1	SUBPROVIDER 2	SUBPROVIDER 3	
GENERAL PATIENT CARE UNITS (EXCLUDING NURSERY) PER DIEM COST				
Total inpatient routine service costs (From line 11, column as appropriate)	$	$	$	44
Total general inpatient routine service cost applicable to Medicare including nursing salary differential adjustment factor (From line 22, column as appropriate)				45
Inpatient routine service cost applicable to outpatient renal dialysis services (From Supplemental Wkst D-7, Part I, column 3, lines 1 and 2 [hospital]; lines 7 and 8 [subprovider I]; lines 9 and 10 [subprovider II])	$	$	$	46
Allowable general inpatient routine service cost subject to apportionment (Line 44 minus sum of lines 45 and 46)				47
Total inpatient days— all patients (From line 3)				48
Inpatient days applicable to title XVIII, Part A (Medicare) (From line 8)				49
Inpatient days applicable to outpatient renal dialysis services (From Supplemental Worksheet D-7, Part I, column 2, lines 1 and 2 [hospital]; lines 7 and 8 [subprovider I]; lines 9 and 10 [subprovider II])				50
Net inpatient days (Line 48 minus sum of lines 49 and 50)				51
Average per diem cost (Line 47 ÷ line 51)	$	$	$	52
NURSERY PER DIEM COST				
Total inpatient cost of nursery (From Worksheet B, column 21, line 51)	$	$	$	53
Total newborn days—nursery (Ff pg 3, Part II, col 1, line 8 [hospital]; pg 4, Part IV, col 1 or col 2, line 8 [subprovider])	$	$	$	54
Average per diem cost—nursery (Line 53 ÷ line 54)	$	$	$	55
GENERAL INPATIENT ROUTINE SERVICE COST				
Inpatient days appl. to title XIX [Ff pg 3, Pt II, col 1, lines 9a [V] or 11a [XIX]; pg 4, Pt IV, col 1, lines 9a [V] or 11a [XIX], as appropriate]	$	$	$	56
General Inpatient routine service cost before reasonable cost limitation (Line 52 × line 56)	$	$	$	57
Title V or title XIX excludable cost (Line 56 × line 32)	$	$	$	58
General inpatient routine service cost for comparison to cost limitation (Line 57 minus line 58)	$	$	$	59
General inpatient routine service cost limitation (Line 56 × $ ___ per diem limitation)	$	$	$	60
Reimbursable general inpatient routine service cost (Line 59 plus the lesser of line 59 or line 60)	$	$	$	61

NURSERY AND INTENSIVE CARE TYPE INPATIENT HOSPITAL UNITS

	TITLE V OR TITLE XIX DAYS 1	AVERAGE PER DIEM (FROM) 2	REIMBURSABLE COSTS (COL. 1 × COL. 2) 3	REIMBURSABLE COSTS (COL. 1 × COL. 2) 4	REIMBURSABLE COSTS (COL. 1 × COL. 2) 5	
Nursery		LINE 35 $	$	$	$	62
Intensive Care Unit		LINE 39 $	$	$	$	63
Coronary Care Unit		LINE 40 $	$	$	$	64
		LINE 41 $	$	$	$	65
		LINE 42 $	$	$	$	66
TOTAL INPATIENT GENERAL ROUTINE, NURSERY AND INTENSIVE CARE TYPE INPATIENT HOSPITAL COSTS (Sum of lines 61–66) (Transfer to Worksheet E-5, Part I, column as appropriate, line 2)		$	$	$	$	67

FORM HCFA-2552-81 (11-81)

28

Exhibit 20

FORM APPROVED
OMB NO. 0938-0050

APPORTIONMENT OF COST OF SERVICES RENDERED BY INTERNS AND RESIDENTS	WORKSHEET D-2

| PROVIDER NO.: | PERIOD: FROM _____ TO _____ | |

PART I — NOT IN APPROVED TEACHING PROGRAM

	COST CENTER	PERCENT OF ASSIGNED TIME	EXPENSE ALLOCATION	TOTAL INPATIENT DAYS—ALL PATIENTS	
		1	2	3	
1	Total cost of services rendered	100 %	$		1
2	Hospital Inpatient Routine Services:				2
3	Adults & Pediatrics (General Routine Care)	%	$		3
4	Intensive Care Unit				4
5	Coronary Care Unit				5
6					6
7					7
8	Nursery				8
9	SUBTOTAL (Sum of lines 3–8)	%	$		9
10	Subprovider I—Inpatient Routine Service				10
11	Subprovider II—Inpatient Routine Service				11
12	Skilled Nursing Facility—Certified				12
13	Skilled Nursing Facility—Noncertified				13
14	Home Health Agency				14
15	SUBTOTAL (Sum of lines 9–14)	%	$		15
				HOSPITAL Total Charges (Fr Wkst C, Col 1, Lines 25 b–27b)	
16	Hospital Outpatient Services:			a	16
17	Clinic	%	$	$	17
18	Emergency				18
19					19
20	SUBTOTAL (Sum of lines 17–19)	%	$		20
21	TOTAL (Sum of lines 15 and 20)	100 %	$		21

PART II — IN AN APPROVED TEACHING PROGRAM (PART B INPATIENT ROUTINE COSTS ONLY)

	COST CENTERS	EXPENSES ALLOCATED TO COST CENTERS ON WKST B, COL 19	
		1	
1	Hospital Inpatient Routine Services:		1
2	Adults & Pediatrics (General Routine Care)	$	2
3	Intensive Care Unit		3
4	Coronary Care Unit		4
5			5
6			6
7	SUBTOTAL (Sum of lines 2–6)	$	7
8	Subprovider I—Inpatient Routine Service		8
9	Subprovider II—Inpatient Routine Service		9
10	Skilled Nursing Facility—Certified		10
11	TOTAL (Sum of lines 7–10)	$	11

PART III — SUMMARY FOR TITLE XVIII (TO BE COMPLETED ONLY IF BOTH PARTS I AND II ARE USED)

		NOT IN APPROVED TEACHING PROGRAM		
	COST CENTERS	REFERENCE (FROM) PART I.	AMOUNT	
		1	2	
1	Hospital			1
2	Inpatient	Col 9, line 9	$	2
3	Outpatient	Col 10, line 20		3
4	TOTAL HOSPITAL (Excluding preadmission diagnostic testing) (Sum of lines 2 and 3)		$	4
5	Hospital outpatient preadmission diagnostic testing	Col 9, line 20	$	5
6	Subprovider I	Col 9, line 10		6
7	Subprovider II	Col 9, line 11		7
8	Skilled Nursing Facility—Certified	Col 9, line 12		8

Exhibit 20 continued

APPORTIONMENT OF COST OF SERVICES RENDERED BY INTERNS AND RESIDENTS	WORKSHEET D-2 Continued

PROVIDER NO.:	PERIOD: FROM ___ TO ___

PART I—NOT IN APPROVED TEACHING PROGRAM

	AVERAGE COST PER DAY (COL 2 − COL 3)	HEALTH CARE PROGRAM INPATIENT DAYS			TITLE V (COL 4 × COL 5)	TITLE XVIII (COL 4 × COL 6)	TITLE XIX (COL 4 × COL 7)	
		TITLE V	TITLE XVIII PART B	TITLE XIX				
	4	5	6	7	8	9	10	
1								1
2								2
3	$				$	$	$	3
4	$							4
5	$							5
6	$							6
7	$							7
8	$							8
9					$	$	$	9
10	$							10
11	$							11
12	$							12
13								13
14								14
15					$	$	$	15

	OUTPATIENT SERVICE CHARGES							
	Pt. B Outpatient 100% Charge (F= Wkst C col 7. lines 25o-27b)	Title XVIII Part B Inpatient Charges (F= Wkst D, cols. 3 & 4 lines 25-27)	Title XVIII Part B 80% Outpatient Charges (F= Wkst C, cols. 8, 9 & 10, lines 25o-27b)	Total Title XVIII Charges (c = d)	Ratio of Cost to Charges (Col 2 − Col e)	Title XVIII Otpt Prand Diag Testing Cost (col. b × col. f)	(col e − col f)	
16	b	c	d	e	f	g	10	16
17	$	$	$	$			$	17
18	$	$	$	$				18
19	$	$	$	$				19
20							$	20
21								21

PART II—IN AN APPROVED TEACHING PROGRAM (PART B INPATIENT ROUTINE COSTS ONLY)

	TOTAL INPATIENT DAYS— ALL PATIENTS	AVERAGE COST PER DAY (COL 1 − COL 2)	TITLE XVIII PART B INPATIENT DAYS	EXPENSES APPLICABLE TO TITLE XVIII (COL 3 × COL 4)	
	2	3	4	5	
1					1
2		$		$	2
3		$			3
4		$			4
5		$			5
6		$			6
7				$	7
8		$			8
9		$			9
10		$			10
11				$	11

PART III — SUMMARY FOR TITLE XVIII (TO BE COMPLETED ONLY IF BOTH PARTS I AND II ARE USED)

	IN APPROVED TEACHING PROGRAM		TOTAL TITLE XVIII COSTS		
	REFERENCE (FROM) PART II. COL. 5 LINE	AMOUNT	REFERENCE (TO) WKST E, PART 1, LINE 4, COL.	AMOUNT (COL 2 − COL 4)	
	3	4	5	6	
1					1
2	7	$		$	2
3					3
4		$	3	$	4
5			2	$	5
6	8		5		6
7	9		7		7
8	10		9		8

Exhibit 21

FORM APPROVED
OMB NO. 0938-0050

APPORTIONMENT OF PROVIDER-BASED PHYSICIAN REMUNERATION FOR PROFESSIONAL SERVICES	WORKSHEET D-3

PROVIDER NO.: _____

PERIOD:
FROM _____
TO _____

PART I—COMBINED BILLING

CHECK ONE:
☐ HOSPITAL   ☐ SUBPROVIDER I   ☐ SUBPROVIDER II

	MEDICAL SPECIALTY DEPARTMENT	TOTAL REMUNERATION APPLICABLE TO PROFESSIONAL SERVICES (1)	TOTAL CHARGES ALL PATIENTS (1)	RATIO OF REMUNERATION TO CHARGES (COL. 1 ÷ COL. 2)	
		1	2	3	
1	RADIOLOGY—DIAGNOSTIC	$	$		1
2	RADIOLOGY—THERAPEUTIC				2
3	RADIOISOTOPE				3
4	PATHOLOGY				4
5	ANESTHESIOLOGY				5
6	ELECTROCARDIOLOGY				6
7	ELECTROENCEPHALOGRAPHY				7
8					8
9					9
10					10
11					11
12	TOTAL (SUM OF LINES 1–11) (2)				12

1	RADIOLOGY—DIAGNOSTIC		1
2	RADIOLOGY—THERAPEUTIC		2
3	RADIOISOTOPE		3
4	PATHOLOGY		4
5	ANESTHESIOLOGY		5
6	ELECTROCARDIOLOGY		6
7	ELECTROENCEPHALOGRAPHY		7
8			8
9			9
10			10
11			11
12	TOTAL (SUM OF LINES 1–11) (2)		12
13	TOTAL NET OF COINSURANCE (LINE 12 × 80%) (3)		13

Exhibit 21 continued

APPORTIONMENT OF PROVIDER-BASED PHYSICIAN REMUNERATION FOR PROFESSIONAL SERVICES	WORKSHEET D-3 Continued

PROVIDER NO.:

PERIOD:
FROM _____
TO _____

PART I—COMBINED BILLING

CHECK ONE: ☐ HOSPITAL   ☐ SUBPROVIDER I   ☐ SUBPROVIDER II

	TITLE V INPATIENT	HEALTH CARE PROGRAM CHARGES					TITLE XIX INPATIENT	INPATIENT/ OUTPATIENT KIDNEY ACQUISITION	
		TITLE XVIII							
		INPATIENT	OUTPATIENT—PART B						
			100%	EMERGENCY SERVICE	ALL OTHER				
	4a	4b	4c	4d	4e		4f	4g	
1	$	$	$	$	$		$	$	1
2									2
3									3
4									4
5									5
6									6
7									7
8									8
9									9
10									10
11									11
12								$	12

	TITLE V INPATIENT	PROFESSIONAL SERVICE REMUNERATION APPLICABLE TO HEALTH CARE PROGRAMS					TITLE XIX INPATIENT	INPATIENT/ OUTPATIENT KIDNEY ACQUISITION	
		TITLE XVIII							
		INPATIENT	OUTPATIENT—PART B						
			100%	EMERGENCY SERVICE	ALL OTHER				
	(COL. 3 × COL. 4a)	(COL. 3 × COL. 4b)	(COL. 3 × COL. 4c)	(COL. 3 × COL. 4d)	(COL. 3 × COL. 4e)		(COL. 3 × COL. 4f)	(COL. 3 × COL. 4g)	
	5a	5b	5c	5d	5e		5f	5g	
1	$	$	$	$	$		$	$	1
2									2
3									3
4									4
5									5
6									6
7									7
8									8
9									9
10									10
11									11
12	$	$	$	$	$		$	$	12
13				$	$				13

(1) If the medical specialty department services the hospital and each subprovider, do not complete columns 1 and 2 on the subprovider worksheets. Enter in column 3 the same ratios developed on the hospital worksheet. If gross combined charges for professional and provider components are used on worksheet C, gross combined charges must be used in column 2 and in columns 4a through 4g. If gross charges for provider component only are used on Worksheet C, gross charges for professional component only must be used in column 2 and in columns 4a through 4g.

(2) Transfer line 12, column:

	TO:
4g	Supplemental Worksheet D-6, Part II, line 2 (Professional Component Charges Only)
5a	Worksheet E-5, Part I, line 11, appropriate column
5b	Worksheet E, Part III, line 57, column 2
5c	Worksheet E, Part III, line 59, column 2
5f	Worksheet E-5, Part I, line 11, appropriate column
5g	Supplemental Worksheet D-6, Part I, line 4, column 3

(3) Transfer line 13, column:

	TO:
5d	Worksheet E, Part III, line 59, column 3, 5, or 7
5e	Worksheet E, Part III, line 59, column 3, 5, or 7

Exhibit 22

FORM APPROVED
OMB NO. 0938-0080

APPORTIONMENT OF PROVIDER-BASED PHYSICIAN REMUNERATION FOR PROFESSIONAL SERVICES	WORKSHEET D-3

PROVIDER NO.: _____

PERIOD:
FROM _____
TO _____

PART II—COMPENSATION-RELATED CHARGE BILLING (OTHER THAN COMBINED BILLING)

CHECK ONE: ☐ HOSPITAL   ☐ SUBPROVIDER I   ☐ SUBPROVIDER II   ☐ SNF

	MEDICAL SPECIALTY DEPARTMENT	TOTAL REMUNERATION APPLICABLE TO PROFESSIONAL SERVICES (1)	TOTAL CHARGES ALL PATIENTS (1)	RATIO OF REMUNERATION TO CHARGES (COL. 1 ÷ COL. 2)	TITLE V INPATIENT	
		1	2	3	4a	
1	RADIOLOGY—DIAGNOSTIC	$	$		$	1
2	RADIOLOGY—THERAPEUTIC					2
3	RADIOISOTOPE					3
4	PATHOLOGY					4
5	ANESTHESIOLOGY					5
6	ELECTROCARDIOLOGY					6
7	ELECTROENCEPHALOGRAPHY					7
8						8
9						9
10						10
11						11
12	TOTAL (SUM OF LINES 1–11) (2)					12

		TITLE V INPATIENT (COL. 3 × COL. 4a)	
		5a	
1	RADIOLOGY—DIAGNOSTIC	$	1
2	RADIOLOGY—THERAPEUTIC		2
3	RADIOISOTOPE		3
4	PATHOLOGY		4
5	ANESTHESIOLOGY		5
6	ELECTROCARDIOLOGY		6
7	ELECTROENCEPHALOGRAPHY		7
8			8
9			9
10			10
11			11
12	TOTAL (SUM OF LINES 1–11) (2)	$	12
13	TOTAL NET OF COINSURANCE (LINE 12 × 80%) (3)		13

Exhibit 22 continued

APPORTIONMENT OF PROVIDER-BASED PHYSICIAN REMUNERATION FOR PROFESSIONAL SERVICES	WORKSHEET D-3 Continued

PROVIDER NO. _____

PERIOD:
FROM _____
TO _____

PART II—COMPENSATION-RELATED CHARGE BILLING (OTHER THAN COMBINED BILLING)

CHECK ONE: ☐ HOSPITAL ☐ SUBPROVIDER I ☐ SUBPROVIDER II ☐ SNF

	HEALTH CARE PROGRAM CHARGES						
	TITLE XVIII					TITLE XIX INPATIENT	INPATIENT/ OUTPATIENT KIDNEY ACQUISITION
	INPATIENT		OUTPATIENT—PART B				
	100%	80%	100%	EMERGENCY SERVICE	ALL OTHER		
	4b	4c	4d	4e	4f	4g	4h
1	$		$	$	$	$	$
2							
3							
4							
5		$					
6							
7							
8							
9							
10							
11							
12							$

	PROFESSIONAL SERVICE REMUNERATION APPLICABLE TO HEALTH CARE PROGRAMS						
	TITLE XVIII					TITLE XIX INPATIENT	INPATIENT/ OUTPATIENT KIDNEY ACQUISITION
	INPATIENT		OUTPATIENT—PART B				
	100% (COL. 3 × COL. 4b)	80% (COL. 3 × COL. 4c)	100% (COL. 3 × COL. 4d)	EMERGENCY SERVICE (COL. 3 × COL. 4e)	ALL OTHER (COL. 3 × COL. 4f)	(COL. 3 × COL. 4g)	(COL. 3 × COL. 4h)
	5b	5c	5d	5e	5f	5g	5h
1	$		$	$	$	$	$
2							
3							
4							
5		$					
6							
7							
8							
9							
10							
11							
12	$	$	$	$	$	$	$
13		$		$	$		

(1) If the medical specialty department services the hospital and each subprovider, do not complete columns 1 and 2 on the subprovider worksheets. Enter in column 3 the same ratios developed on the hospital worksheet.

(2) Transfer the amounts on line 12, column(s):

	TO:
4h	Supplemental Worksheet D-6, Part II, line 2 (Professional Component Charges Only)
5e and 5g	The respective title V and title XIX Worksheet E-5, Part I, line 11
5b	Worksheet E, Part III, line 58, column 2
5d	Worksheet E, Part III, line 60, column 2
5h	Supplemental Worksheet D-6, Part I, line 4

(3) Transfer the amounts on line 13, column(s):

	TO:
5c	Worksheet E, Part III, line 58, column 3, 5, 7, or 9 as appropriate
5e and 5f	Worksheet E, Part III, line 60, column 3, 5, 7, or 9 as appropriate

FORM HCFA-2552-81 (11-81)

31 Continued

Exhibit 23

FORM APPROVED
OMB NO. 0938-0050

APPORTIONMENT OF MALPRACTICE INSURANCE COSTS	PROVIDER NO.:		PERIOD: FROM _____ TO _____		WORKSHEET D-8

	PART 1—PAID MALPRACTICE LOSSES	TITLE V	TITLE XVIII	TITLE XIX	OTHER	TOTAL (Sum of cols 1-4)
		1	2	3	4	5
1	Current period losses	$	$	$	$	$
2	PRIOR PERIOD LOSSES: Cost reporting period ended: 19 __					
3	19 __					
4	19 __					
5	19 __					
6	Total (Sum of lines 1-5)	$	$	$	$	$

PART II—APPORTIONMENT TO HEALTH CARE PROGRAMS

7	If there are no entries on lines 1 through 6, enter the national ratio for:			
	a. TITLE V _____		b. TITLE XVIII _____	c. TITLE XIX _____

	If line 7 is completed DO NOT complete lines 8, 9 and 10		
8	Ratio of title V malpractice losses to total (col 1, line 6 ÷ col 5, line 6)		
9	Ratio of title XVIII malpractice losses to total (col 2, line 6 ÷ col 5, line 6)		
10	Ratio of title XIX malpractice losses to total (col 3, line 6 ÷ col 5, line 6)		
11	Current period malpractice insurance premiums or fund contrib.'s (See instructions)		$
12	Home health agency malpractice insurance premiums and/or fund contributions		
	From Wkst B, col 21, sum of lines 60-67 plus Wkst C, col. 15, line 30a $ _____ — _____ × line 11		( )
	From Wkst B, col 21, line 79 $ _____		
13	Net malpractice insurance premiums and/or fund contributions (line 11 minus line 12)		$
14	Total title V malpractice insurance costs (line 7a or 8 × line 13)		$
15	Total title XVIII malpractice insurance costs (line 7b or 9 × line 13)		$
16	Total title XIX malpractice insurance costs (line 7c or 10 × line 13)		$

	DESCRIPTION	HEALTH CARE (1) PROGRAM CHARGES	RATIO (2)	COST (3)
		1	2	3
17	TITLE V			
a	Hospital	$		$
b	Subprovider I			
c	Subprovider II			
d	Total title V charges	$	1.00000000	$
18	TITLE XVIII			
a	Hospital—Part A	$		$
b	Hospital—Part B—100%			
c	Hospital—Part B—80%			
d	Subprovider I—Part A			
e	Subprovider I—Part B			
f	Subprovider II—Part A			
g	Subprovider II—Part B			
h	Skilled Nursing Facility—Part A			
i	Skilled Nursing Facility—Part B			
j	Total title XVIII charges	$	1.00000000	$
19	TITLE XIX			
a	Hospital	$		$
b	Subprovider I			
c	Subprovider II			
d	Total title XIX charges	$	1.00000000	$

PART III—DIRECTLY ASSIGNED MALPRACTICE COSTS—TITLE V AND TITLE XIX

		TITLE V	TITLE XIX
		1	2
20	Hospital (See Instructions)	$	$
21	Subprovider I (See Instructions)	$	$
22	Subprovider II (See Instructions)	$	$

PART IV—DIRECTLY ASSIGNED MALPRACTICE COSTS—TITLE XVIII

		PART A	PART B-100%	PART B-80%
		1	2	3
23	HOSPITAL	$	$	$
24	SUBPROVIDER I	$		$
25	SUBPROVIDER II	$		$
26	SKILLED NURSING FACILITY	$		$

(1) Title XVIII Charges—From Worksheet E, Part II, columns 1-9, line 43, Titles V and XIX Charges—From the appropriate Worksheet E-5, Part II, columns 1-3, line 32.
(2) Divide each component's health care program charges by its total health care program charges for title V, title XVIII and title XIX.
(3) To obtain cost, multiply the ratios in column 2, times line 14 (title V), line 15 (title XVIII), line 16 (title XIX).

Medicare Regulations Regarding Hospital Reimbursement

The following Medicare instructions apply, at this writing, to the determination of hospital reimbursement, as discussed in Chapter 8. Relevant worksheets, identified by exhibit number from the list at the end of this Appendix, are included. Techniques to determine reimbursement are applied to the statistical schedule as well as on Medicare Worksheet E through Worksheet G-5.

If appropriate, enter on line 6, the kidney acquisition costs applicable to patients covered under title V or title XIX, but who are not covered under title XVIII. The costs should be determined in the manner described in the instructions for Worksheet E, Part I, line 16.

Line 8--Enter in the appropriate column the applicable charge differential between semiprivate and less than semiprivate accommodations. The amount of the differential is the difference between the provider's customary charge for the less than semiprivate accommodations and its customary charge for the accommodations furnished for all health care program patient days where the accommodations furnished were provided not at the patient's request, nor for a reason which is consistent with health care program purposes.

Line 10--Enter in the appropriate columns the professional remuneration paid to hospital-based physicians for inpatient services rendered to health care program beneficiaries. These lines will be completed only when combined billing is used.

Line 11--Enter any amounts paid and payable by workers' compensation. Such amounts should be for the cost of services which is included in the health care program's share of allowable costs. Generally, such amounts are applicable to routine services.

346.2   Part II - Computation of the Lesser of Reasonable Cost or Customary Charges.--Providers will be paid the lesser of the reasonable cost of services furnished to beneficiaries or the customary charges made by the provider for the same services. This part provides for the computation of the lesser of reasonable cost as defined in Health Insurance Regulations section 405.455 (b)(2) or customary charges as defined in Health Insurance Regulations section 405.455(b)(1).

LINE DESCRIPTIONS

Lines 1 through 4--These lines provide for the computation of reasonable cost of inpatient services applicable to the health care program.

Lines 5 through 10--These lines provide for the accumulation of charges which relate to the reasonable cost on line 4.

Do not include on these lines the portion of charges applicable to the excess costs of luxury items or services (see PRM, Part I, chapter 21).

Enter on line 6, the health care program charges for inpatient ancillary services. If the charges on Worksheet D do not include the professional component of   hospital-based physician remuneration, the amount to be entered on line 6 should be obtained from the appropriate Worksheet D, columns 2 or 5, line 28. However, if the charges on Worksheet D do include such professional component, the amount of the professional component should be eliminated from the charges to be entered on line 6.

The amounts entered on line 7 should include covered late charges which have been billed to the health care program where the patient's medical condition is the cause of the stay past the checkout time. Also, these amounts should include charges relating to a stay in a special care unit for a few hours where the provider's normal practice is to bill for the partial stay. In addition, these charges should include the semi-private charges of accommodations of health care program inpatients for which workers' compensation was paid at the rate of the ward accommodation charges and for which the workers' compensation payment will subsequently be deducted from final settlement.

Lines 11 through 15--These lines provide for the appropriate reduction of charges where the provider does not actually impose such charges in the case of most patients liable for payment for services on a charge basis or fails to make reasonable efforts to collect such charges from those patients. Providers which do impose these charges and make reasonable efforts to collect the charges from patients liable for payment for services on a charge basis are not required to complete lines 11 through 14, but should enter on line 15, the amount from line 10. See Health Insurance Regulations section 405.455(b).

In no instance may the customary charges on line 15 exceed the actual charges on line 10.

346.3 Part III - Computation of Reimbursement Settlement.--

LINE DESCRIPTIONS

Line 7--Enter on this line the program's share of any net depreciation adjustment applicable to prior years resulting from the gain or loss on the disposition of depreciable assets (see PRM, Part I, chapter 1). Enter the amount of any excess depreciation taken in parenthesis (   ).

Line 8--Enter on this line the Medicare program's share of any recovery of excess depreciation applicable to prior years resulting from provider termination of a decrease in Medicare utilization (see PRM, Part I, chapter 1).

348. WORKSHEET G - BALANCE SHEET

348.1 Worksheet G-1 - Statement of Charges in Fund Balances.--

348.2 Worksheet G-2 - Statement of Patient Revenues and Operating Expenses.--

384.3 Worksheet G-3 - Statement of Revenue and Expenses.--These worksheets are to be prepared from the provider's accounting books and records. Additional worksheets may be submitted, if necessary.

Worksheets G and G-1 are to be completed by all providers maintaining fund-type accounting records. Nonproprietary providers, not maintaining fund-type accounting records, should complete the "General Fund" columns only.

Proprietary providers not maintaining fund-type accounting records should not complete Worksheet G since such providers will have already completed Supplemental Worksheet F, Part I (Balance Sheet for Computation of Equity Capital). Also, these providers should complete the "General Fund" column only on Worksheet G-1. Worksheets G-2 and G-3 must be completed by all providers.

The provider may substitute its own financial statements for these forms provided the information shown on such statements is at least as detailed as that requested on the HCFA forms.

Supplemental Worksheets
(Available Upon Request From Intermediary)

350. SUPPLEMENTAL WORKSHEET D-4 - APPORTIONMENT OF REMUNERATION APPLICABLE TO HOSPITAL-BASED PATHOLOGISTS FOR PROFESSIONAL SERVICES REIMBURSABLE UNDER PART A AND FURNISHED UNDER ARRANGEMENTS BY THE HOSPITAL TO THE HOSPITAL-BASED SKILLED NURSING FACILITY INPATIENTS

When hospital-based skilled nursing facility inpatients receive laboratory services from the hospital, such services are considered to be provided under arrangements with the hospital so that the usual rules in regard to laboratory services provided under arrangements by one provider for the inpatients of another are applicable, i.e., the entire service is covered as a provider service under Part A. Therefore, it is necessary to separately determine what portion of the pathologists' remuneration for personal patient care services which was eliminated from allowable cost on Worksheet A-8, column 2, line 9, is applicable to the laboratory services furnished to the hospital-based skilled nursing facility Medicare inpatients and include that amount as part of the hospital-based skilled nursing facility's Part A reimbursable cost.

This worksheet provides for the calculation of the hospital-based pathologists' remuneration applicable to services rendered under arrangements by the hospital to Medicare inpatients of the hospital-based skilled nursing facility.

Providers billing on behalf of the pathologists for professional services under the form HCFA-1554 billing procedure should complete lines 1 and 2 in order to compute the ratio of the remuneration for professional services rendered by pathologists to total charges - all patients for the pathology department. Providers billing for patient services by pathologists under combined billing should not complete lines 1 and 2. The ratio of total remuneration to total charges to be entered on line 3 should be obtained from Worksheet D-3, column 3, line 4.

355.   SUPPLEMENTAL WORKSHEET D-5 - COST APPORTIONMENT OF
        AMBULANCE SERVICES RENDERED BY PROVIDER
Ambulance services rendered to inpatients covered under titles V, XVIII and XIX and rendered to outpatients covered under title XVIII are reimbursable by the respective health care programs. Such services rendered to title XVIII (Medicare) patients are reimbursable, subject to the deductible and coinsurance amounts, only on behalf of individuals enrolled under Part B. (See PRM, Part I, chapter 21.)

360.   SUPPLEMENTAL WORKSHEET D-6 - COMPUTATION OF KIDNEY
        ACQUISITION COSTS AND CHARGES - SUPPLEMENTARY TO INPATIENT
        ROUTINE AND INPATIENT ANCILLARY SERVICE COSTS AND CHARGES
The total inpatient routine cost apportioned to Medicare on Worksheet D-1 and the total inpatient ancillary cost apportioned to Medicare on Worksheet D include the total of such costs applicable to kidney acquisitions. This worksheet provides for the computation and accumulation of the balance of the provider's costs which are applicable to kidney acquisitions and which are to be included in Medicare costs.

The use of this worksheet is optional. It will not be completed when the provider elects to be reimbursed for kidney acquisition costs under the ALTERNATIVE PROCEDURES. If the provider has elected to be reimbursed under the ALTERNATIVE PROCEDURES, the costs otherwise accumulated on this worksheet will be treated in the following manner:

    A.   Kidney Acquisition Outpatient Costs.--To avoid the need for separate reimbursement settlement, the charges generated in the rendition of kidney acquisition hospital outpatient services will be included with hospital inpatient charges on Worksheet C, column 3, and excluded from outpatient charges on Worksheet C, columns 7 through 9. These charges will also be included with Medicare inpatient charges on Worksheet D, column 3.

B. Kidney Acquisition Services Rendered By Interns and
Residents Not In Approved Teaching Program.

Inpatient--Kidney acquisition inpatient days will be included with
Medicare Part B inpatient days on Worksheet D-2, Part I, column 6.

Outpatient--Kidney acquisition outpatient charges were included
with Medicare inpatient charges (see item A above). Therefore,
under the ALTERNATIVE PROCEDURES, these charges will not be part
of outpatient charges used to apportion such cost to the program
on Worksheet D-2, Part I, lines 17 through 19.

C. Kidney Acquisition Costs Applicable to Professional
Remuneration of Hospital-Based Physicians Under Combined Billing.--
If the provider and the physician agree, the provider component
and professional component split of the physician remuneration may
be adjusted to include a higher portion in provider costs. This
higher portion must be directly related to the amount of time the
physicians spend on kidney acquisition services. The intermediary
and carrier must agree to the additional amount applicable to
such kidney acquisition services and to the corresponding reduction which must be made to the Part B physician charges. In this
case, the adjustment on Worksheet A-8, lines 8 through 12, as
appropriate, will reflect the reduced amount of the physician
component. Also, if the combined billing procedure is used, the
kidney acquisition charges should be eliminated from the total
charges and kidney acquisition charges which would otherwise have
been used in the apportionment computation of the physicians'
professional remuneration on Worksheet D-3.

D. Direct Kidney Acquisition Costs.--The provider should
include these costs in the various provider department cost
centers, as appropriate.

360.1 Part I - Computation of Kidney Acquisition Costs (Other
Than Inpatient Routine and Inpatient Ancillary Service Costs).--

Lines 1a through 1f--These lines are used to apportion to the
program the cost of inpatient services attributable to kidney
acquisitions rendered in each of the inpatient routine areas by
interns and residents not in an approved teaching program.

Column 1--Enter on the appropriate lines the average per
diem cost of interns and residents not in an approved
teaching program in each of the inpatient routine areas.
These amounts are obtained from Worksheet D-2, Part I,
column 4, line as indicated.

Column 2--Enter the number of kidney acquisition days in
each of the inpatient routine areas from page 2, Part II,
line 10h, or page 3, Part IV, line 10h.

Column 3--Multiply the per diem amount in column 1 by the
number of days in column 2.

Line 2--These lines provide for the computation of the cost of
outpatient services attributable to kidney acquisitions rendered in
each of the outpatient service areas by interns and residents not
in an approved teaching program.

Column 1--Enter on the appropriate lines the kidney acquisition
charges in each of the outpatient service areas. These amounts
are obtained from Worksheet C, column 8, line as indicated.

Column 2--Enter the ratio of the outpatient cost of interns
and residents not in an approved teaching program to the
hospital outpatient service charges in each of the outpatient
service areas. These ratios are obtained from Worksheet D-2,
Part I, column e, line as indicated.

Column 3--Multiply the charge in column 1 by the ratio in
column 2.

Line 3--Enter the kidney acquisition cost of hospital outpatient
services from Worksheet C, column 8, line 34a.

Line 4--Enter on this line the remuneration for professional
services rendered by hospital-based physicians under combined billing
and which are applicable to kidney acquisitions. This amount is
obtained from Worksheet D-3, column 5e, line 12.

Line 5--Enter the direct kidney acquisition costs from Worksheet B,
column 21, line 42.

These direct costs include, but are not limited to, the costs of
services purchased under arrangements or billed directly to the
provider for:

        a. Fees for physician services (pre-admission donor and
recipient tissue typing).

        b. Costs for kidneys acquired from other providers or
kidney procurement organizations.

        c. Transportation costs of kidneys.

        d. Kidney recipient registration fees.

        e. Surgeons' fees for excising cadaveric kidneys.

        f. Tissue typing services furnished by independent
laboratories.

Line 6--Enter the sum of lines 1f and 2d through 5. This amount
constitutes the provider's total kidney acquisition cost in addition to the inpatient routine and inpatient ancillary service costs,
which were apportioned with and included in Medicare inpatient
costs. Transfer this amount to Worksheet E, Part I, line 8.

360.2 Part II - Computation of Kidney Acquisition Charges (Other
Than Inpatient Routine and Inpatient Ancillary Service Charges).--
This part provides for the accumulation of the charges which relate to
the costs on Part I, line 6. These charges will be added to
Medicare charges on Worksheet E, Part II, for comparison with
reasonable cost as provided in Health Insurance Regulations
section 405.455.

Line 1--Enter on this line the kidney acquisition outpatient
charges. If the charges on Worksheet C, column 8, line 34b,
include charges for provider component only, such charges should
be entered on this line. Otherwise, the professional component
should be eliminated from the amount on Worksheet C, column 8,
line 34b, before transferring to this line.

Line 2--Enter on this line that part of the kidney acquisition
charges in all departments for which combined billing is used
(from Worksheet D-3, column 4e, line 12) which represents the
charges for the physician remuneration for professional services.
If gross combined charges are used on Worksheet D-3, the provider
component of such charges must be removed before transferring the
amount in column 4e, line 12, to this line.

Line 3--If the provider has a schedule of charges which represents
the various direct kidney acquisition costs included in Part I,
line 5 (i.e., costs for kidneys acquired from others, transporta-
tion, etc.), enter on this line the total of the charges which
are applicable to the costs in Part I, line 5. However, if the
provider has no such schedule of charges, enter on this line the
amount in Part I, line 5.

Line 4--Enter the sum of lines 1 through 3. This amount constitutes
the charges for kidney acquisition services in addition to the
inpatient routine and inpatient ancillary service charges. Transfer this amount to Worksheet E, Part II, line 12.

360.3 Part III - Other Data.--The data to be entered in this part
are data applicable to all components of the health care complex.

Lines 1a, 1b and 1c--Indicate on the appropriate line the number
of kidneys transplanted by this provider in Medicare patients (1a),
in non-Medicare patients (1b) and in all provider patients (1c).
The sum of lines 1a and 1b should be entered on line 1c.

Line 2--Enter the total number of kidneys furnished to other
providers, kidney procurement organizations or others. Such
kidneys need not have been furnished for transplant purposes.

Line 3--Enter the total number of kidneys which were not suitable
for transplant or which were used for other purposes within this
provider.

Line 4--Enter the total number of kidneys which were excised
within this provider or which were acquired from other providers
or kidney procurement organizations. This total should agree
with the sum of the number of kidneys on lines 1c through 3.

Line 5--Enter the number of kidneys transplanted by the provider
into non-Medicare patients, and kidneys furnished to others for
which revenue on Worksheet E, Part I, line 16, was received.

365.   SUPPLEMENTAL WORKSHEET D-7 - ADJUSTMENT TO RENAL DIALYSIS
        COST CENTER FOR PROVIDERS USING ACCOMMODATIONS OTHER THAN
        IN THE DIALYSIS DEPARTMENT TO FURNISH RENAL DIALYSIS SERVICES
This worksheet is to be prepared only by providers that furnished
outpatient renal dialysis services and used either an inpatient
routine bed and/or a bed or other accommodation in the outpatient
areas (other than in the dialysis department) in order to furnish
this service. For example, an inpatient routine bed which is
physically outside the renal dialysis department is sometimes
used to accommodate a patient who receives peritoneal renal dialysis,
and the length of time for the treatment exceeds approximately
30 hours. If the provider furnishes renal dialysis in the
dialysis department (in the manner in which such service is
typically furnished), this worksheet is to give recognition to the costs
incurred by providers in utilizing either inpatient beds, or beds
or other accommodations in the provider's outpatient department
(other than in the dialysis department) to furnish outpatient
renal dialysis. Such costs, including overhead, must be transferred to the renal dialysis cost center after cost finding. Of
course, where beds or other accommodations within the renal
dialysis department are utilized, all appropriate costs have been
recognized in the renal dialysis cost center through the cost
finding process.

365.1 Part I - Computation of Inpatient Routine Service Cost
Applicable to Renal Dialysis.--This part is to be completed only
by providers that used inpatient routine beds to furnish outpatient
renal dialysis services.

Column 1--Enter the per diem costs from the indicated lines of
the appropriate Worksheet D-1.

Column 2--Enter the number of inpatient days applicable to outpatient renal dialysis. In counting renal dialysis days, one-half day is counted for each renal dialysis session (either hemodialysis or peritoneal dialysis) that does not exceed 12 hours duration. If a treatment exceeds 12 hours duration, a full day is counted unless the treatment is of such duration that more than one inpatient day could be counted under the customary procedures for counting inpatient days, in which case the customary procedures for counting inpatient days will prevail. However, not more than one inpatient day can be counted for any bed on the same calendar day. For example, if two different renal dialysis patients occupied the same bed at different times during one calendar day, only one renal dialysis day would be counted.

Column 3--Compute the amount of inpatient routine cost applicable to outpatient renal dialysis by multiplying the per diem cost in column 1 by the number of renal dialysis days in column 2.

365.2 Part II - Computation of Outpatient Service Cost Applicable To Renal Dialysis.--This part is to be completed only by providers that used beds or other accommodations in the outpatient area (outside the renal dialysis department) in furnishing outpatient renal dialysis.

Column 1--Enter the total outpatient service charges for each outpatient service area (excluding charges for renal dialysis) applicable to renal dialysis patients for use of an outpatient bed or other accommodation. This amount should be obtained from the provider's records.

Column 2--Enter in this column the ratio of total cost to total charges for each outpatient service cost center. These ratios are obtained from Worksheet C, column 2, line as indicated.

Column 3--Compute the outpatient cost applicable to renal dialysis by multiplying the charges in column 1 by the ratios in column 2.

365.3 Part III - Computation of Adjusted Renal Dialysis Cost.-- Compute the adjusted renal dialysis cost in accordance with the line descriptions on this part and transfer this amount to Worksheet C, column 1, line 21a.

370. SUPPLEMENTAL WORKSHEET E-3 - APPLICATION OF THE LIMITATION
      ON OUTPATIENT RENAL DIALYSIS COSTS
The purpose of this worksheet is to apply the limitations for the cost of outpatient maintenance renal dialysis services (including both hemodialysis and peritoneal dialysis) and training self dialysis sessions.

The limitation is not applied to providers that do not regularly
furnish outpatient routine maintenance dialysis services.
Providers that furnish outpatient renal dialysis services on an
emergency basis only, or infrequently as a maintenance service,
should not complete this worksheet. Also, the limitation does
not apply to dialysis services furnished to inpatients who are
institutionalized for a medical reason other than to receive
maintenance dialysis (e.g., tonsillectomy).

Providers which furnish hemodialysis and peritoneal dialysis may
be subject to a separate limit for each of the two types of
service. If hemodialysis is usually furnished in six-hour sessions
three times a week and peritoneal dialysis is furnished in ten-hour
sessions two times a week, separate limits may be appropriate.
However, if both types of service are furnished in comparable
time frames and frequencies, one limit may be applicable to both
services. In this latter situation, both types of services should
be entered in column 1.

Explanations are provided for the following lines.

Line 3--For each type of outpatient dialysis service, enter from
the provider records the total Medicare charges for the renal
dialysis related routine laboratory services performed in the
hospital's laboratory or in another laboratory under arrangements.
These routine laboratory services were considered in the determination of the interim renal dialysis screens which were furnished
to the provider by the intermediary.

NOTE: If all of the related routine laboratory services
        are performed by a certified independent laboratory or
        another hospital laboratory, and such other laboratory
        bills its Part B carrier or its intermediary directly
        for such services, lines 3 and 4 need not be completed.
        In this situation, the interim renal dialysis screen
        should have been adjusted accordingly.

Line 9--Enter the applicable limitation. Unless a different cost
limitation has been approved by the Department of Health and Human
Services, the applicable limitations are: $145.00 for each out-
patient routine maintenance dialysis (either hemodialysis or
peritoneal dialysis) exclusive of the routine laboratory services
associated with the dialysis; $150.00 for each outpatient
maintenance dialysis session (either hemodialysis or peritoneal
dialysis) if the related routine laboratory services are included
in the cost; $185.00 for a self training dialysis session exclusive
of the related routine laboratory services; and $190.00 for a self
training dialysis session if the related routine laboratory
services are included in the cost. However, for services
rendered after June 30, 1974, the cost limitations for self training
dialysis sessions are $165.00 and $170.00, respectively. With

respect to outpatient peritoneal dialysis extended sessions of at
least 30-hours duration, the cost limitation is $435.00 for each
extended session exclusive of the related routine laboratory services,
and $450.00 for each extended session if the related routine labora-
tory services are included in the cost. In all cases, the costs
will not include the routine laboratory cost when it is not
necessary to complete lines 3 and 4 in accordance with the instructions.

Line 10--Compute the total cost limitation for each specified type
of dialysis service by multiplying the number of sessions on line 8
by the amount on line 9. If more than one limitation for a type
of renal dialysis service is applicable during a cost reporting
period, the amount of total cost limitation must be computed by
taking all unit cost limitations into account to the extent that
each limitation was applicable during the cost reporting period.
This will be accomplished by adding the amounts determined by
multiplying each unit cost limitation applicable during the cost
reporting period by the number of sessions furnished during the
period that the limitation was applicable. Providers should add
a worksheet to the cost report showing this computation.

Line 11--Compute the excess of actual costs over the maximum
limitations by subtracting the amount on line 10 from the amount
on line 7 in each column. If in any column, the amount on line 7
is equal to or less than the amount on line 10, enter zero on
line 11 of that column, and do not complete line 12 in that column.

375. SUPPLEMENTAL WORKSHEET E-4 - RECOVERY OF UNREIMBURSED COST -
      OTHER THAN NEW PROVIDERS
This worksheet should not be completed by a public provider which
renders services free of charge or at a nominal charge. (See PRM,
Part I, chapter 26.)

A separate copy of this worksheet should be completed for each
health care program under which costs are unreimbursed or recovery
of previously unreimbursed cost is requested by "other than new
providers." Also, a separate copy of this worksheet should be
completed for each "other than new provider" component of a health
care complex, as appropriate.

This worksheet should be used by "other than a new provider" to
accumulate unreimbursed cost and to compute the recovery of
previously unreimbursed cost under Health Insurance Regulations
Section 405.455 (Lesser of Cost or Charges).

For purposes of using this worksheet, "other than new providers"
refers to a provider which has operated as the type of facility
(or the equivalent thereof) for which it is certified in the
health care program under present or previous ownership for 3 full
years or more and which is not currently operating within the new
provider recovery period. EXCEPTION: An "other than new provider"

should also use this worksheet if it is operating within the new provider recovery period, but it is not carrying forward any cost previously unreimbursed within the new provider base period. See the Health Insurance Regulations sections 405.455 and 405.460.

A new provider should, in lieu of this worksheet, use Supplemental Worksheet E-4-1, which can be obtained from your intermediary.

Titles V and XIX recovery computation will be completed using the Part A column only.

375.1 Part I - Computation of Recovery of Unreimbursed Cost Under Lesser of Cost or Charges.--Part A, column 1, should not be completed in any cost reporting period in which costs are unreimbursed under Health Insurance Regulations Section 405.460 (Limitations on Coverage of Costs). See Worksheet D-1, Part I, lines 23 through 39 and Part II, lines 57 through 62.

375.2 Part II - Computation of Carryover of Unreimbursed Cost Under Lesser of Cost or Charges.--

Line 1--If the amounts entered on the prior year's cost report Supplemental Worksheet E-4, Part II, columns 5 through 8, line 4, represent cost reporting periods which, when combined, contain at least 24 full calendar months, then such amounts should be entered in columns 3 through 6, line 1, respectively. However, if such combined cost reporting periods contain fewer than 24 full calendar months, the amounts entered on Supplemental Worksheet E-4, Part II, columns 3 through 8, line 4, of the prior year's cost report should be entered in columns 1 through 6, line 1.

NOTE: However, for the prior year cost reporting period which
        began before July 1, 1979, the amounts to be entered on
        line 1 are determined as follows: Multiply the amount
        from the prior year's cost report Supplemental
        Worksheet E-4, Part II, column as appropriate, line 4,
        by the ratios from Worksheet E, Part II, column as
        appropriate, line 6, for the cost reporting period in
        which the costs were unreimbursed.

Line 2--The total amount of unreimbursed cost recovered in the current cost reporting period and to be entered in columns 9 and 10 should be obtained from Part I, line 3. The recovery of unreimbursed cost applicable to each cost reporting period (columns 1 through 6) in which a carryover of previously unreimbursed cost exists will be made on a first-in - first-out basis. That is, the recovery should first be applied to columns 1 and/or 2, then to columns 3 and/or 4, etc. The amounts entered on line 2 may not exceed the amounts on line 1 in any column.

Line 3--Enter in columns 7 and 8, the amount obtained from
Worksheet E, Part II, line 24, or Worksheet E-5, Part II, line 17,
whichever is appropriate. If any amount is entered on line 2,
enter zero on line 3.

380.   SUPPLEMENTAL WORKSHEET E-4-1 - RECOVERY OF UNREIMBURSED
       COST - NEW PROVIDERS
A separate copy of this worksheet should be completed for each
health care program under which costs are unreimbursed or recovery
of previously unreimbursed cost is requested by a "new provider."
Also, a separate copy of this worksheet should be completed for
each "new provider" component of a health care complex, as
appropriate.

A new provider is an institution that has operated as the type of
facility (or the equivalent thereof) for which it is certified
in the program under present and previous ownership for less than
3 full years.

This worksheet should be used by a new provider to accumulate
unreimbursed cost under Health Insurance Regulations Section
405.455 (Lesser of Cost or Charges) and to compute the recovery
of previously unreimbursed cost under Health Insurance Regulations
Sections 405.455 (Lesser of Cost or Charges) and 405.460 (Limitations on Coverage of Costs) during both the new provider base
period and the new provider recovery period.

That is, a new provider should continue to complete this
worksheet until all costs which were unreimbursed during the
new provider base period are recovered or the new provider recovery
period ends, whichever occurs first. Thereafter, Supplemental
Worksheet E-4, which can be obtained from your intermediary,
should be used in lieu of this worksheet, if necessary.

The new provider base period is any cost reporting period under
which costs are reimbursed under Health Insurance Regulations
sections 405.455 and 405.460 and which end on or before the last
day of the new provider's third year of operation.

The new provider recovery period is the five cost reporting
periods immediately succeeding the new provider base period. If
the five succeeding cost reporting periods combined include fewer
than 60 full calendar months, the new provider may carry forward
such unreimbursed cost for one additional reporting period.

Titles V and XIX recovery computation will be completed using the
Part A column only.

380.1 Part I - Computation of Recovery of Unreimbursed Cost.--
Part I is provided for the computation of the recovery of
unreimbursed cost under Health Insurance Regulations Section

405.455 (Lesser of Cost or Charges) and previously unreimbursed
cost under Health Insurance Regulations Section 405.460
(Limitations on Coverage of Costs).

This part should not be completed for a provider in any cost
reporting period in which costs are unreimbursed under
section 405.455. Also, Part A, column 1, should not be completed
for a provider in any cost reporting period in which costs are
unreimbursed under section 405.460. Even though customary
charges exceed reasonable cost, a provider is prohibited from
recovering previously unreimbursed costs under section 405.455
whenever costs are unreimbursed under section 405.460 during the
same cost reporting period.

Also, when reasonable cost equals or exceeds customary charges,
the provider is prohibited from recovering previously unreimbursed
cost under both sections 405.455 and 405.460.

SPECIAL INSTRUCTIONS FOR PUBLIC PROVIDERS WHICH RENDER SERVICES
FREE OF CHARGE OR AT A NOMINAL CHARGE

Public providers rendering services free of charge or at a
nominal charge are not subject to the lesser of cost or charges
provisions. (See PRM, Part I, chapter 26.) These providers
should not complete lines 1, 4 and 5. The recovery of unreimbursed cost under cost limits to be entered on line 3 will be
line 2.

380.2 Part II - Computation of Carryover of Unreimbursed Cost
Under Cost Limits.--This part is provided for the computation of
the carryover of previously unreimbursed cost under section
405.460. New providers only may carry forward to subsequent
cost reporting periods (New Provider Recovery Period) previously
unreimbursed cost from the new provider base period.

Line 3--The carryover at the end of the current cost reporting
period will be the beginning carryover (line 1) for the following
period.

380.3 Part III - Computation of Carryover of Unreimbursed Cost
Under Lesser of Cost or Charges.--Public providers rendering
services free of charge or at a nominal charge should not
complete this part.

Line 1--The amounts entered in columns 1 through 8, line 1 should
be obtained as follows:

    1. The amounts to be entered in columns 1 and 2 should be
obtained from the prior year's cost report Supplemental Worksheet
E-4-1, Part III, columns 1 and 2, line 4.

NOTE: However, for prior year cost reporting periods which began
       before July 1, 1979, providers which have more than one
       cost reporting period in the new provider base period
       should compute the Part A and Part B columns as follows:

380.3(Cont.)   FORM HCFA-2552   8-80

     1. For column 1, multiply the amount from the prior
year's cost report Supplemental Worksheet E-4-1, Part III,
column 1, line 4, by the cumulative ratio of total Part A cost to
total cost for all cost reporting periods in which costs were
unreimbursed in the new provider base period.

     2. For column 2, multiply the amount from the prior
year's cost report Supplemental Worksheet E-4-1, Part III,
column 1, line 4, by the cumulative ratio of total Part B cost
to total cost for all cost reporting periods in which costs were
unreimbursed in the new provider base period.

     2. If the amounts entered on the prior year's cost report
Supplemental Worksheet E-4-1, Part III, columns 7 through 10,
line 4, represent cost reporting periods which, when combined,
contain at least 24 full calendar months, then such amounts should
be entered in columns 5 through 8, line 1, respectively. However,
if such combined cost reporting periods contain fewer than 24 full
calendar months, the amounts entered on Supplemental Worksheet
E-4-1, Part III, columns 5 through 10, line 4 of the prior year's
cost report should be entered in columns 3 through 8, line 1.

NOTE: However, for the prior year cost reporting period which
      began before July 1, 1979, the amounts to be entered on
      line 1 are determined as follows: Multiply the amount
      from the prior year's cost report Supplemental Work-
      sheet E-4-1, Part III, column as appropriate, line 4,
      by the ratios from Worksheet E, Part II, column as
      appropriate, line 6, for the cost reporting period in
      which the costs were unreimbursed.

Line 2--The total amount of unreimbursed cost recovered in the
current cost reporting period and to be entered in columns 11 and
12 should be obtained from Part I, line 5, columns 1 and 2.

The recovery of unreimbursed cost applicable to each cost
reporting period (columns 1 through 8) in which a carryover of
previously reimbursed cost exists will be made on a first-in -
first-out basis. That is, the recovery should first be applied
to columns 1 and/or 2 then to columns 3 and/or 4, etc. The
amounts entered on line 2 may not exceed the amounts on line 1 in
any column.

Exception to the first-in - first-out basis for recovery of
previously disallowed cost: If under section 223 a provider has
cost disallowed in its first or second cost reporting period of
the new provider recovery period, it should compute the recovery
of these disallowed costs in columns 3 through 8 before computing
any recovery applicable to the base period in columns 1 and 2.
Of course, the first-in - first-out basis should be used with

respect to columns 3 through 8. The reason for this exception
is because the recovery period for costs disallowed in the first
and second cost reporting period of the recovery period will
expire prior to the recovery period for costs disallowed in the
new provider base period.

Line 3--Columns 1 and 2 will be completed only when there is
unreimbursed cost attributable to the current cost reporting
period and the current cost reporting period is also included
within the new provider base period.

Columns 9 and 10 will be used whenever there is unreimbursed cost
in the current cost reporting period which is within the new
provider recovery period. Columns 9 and 10 will not be used when
the current cost reporting period is within the new provider base
period.

If any amount is entered on line 2, enter zero in the appropriate
column on line 3.

385. SUPPLEMENTAL WORKSHEET F - RETURN ON EQUITY CAPITAL OF
      PROPRIETARY PROVIDERS
This worksheet provides for the calculation of a reasonable return
on equity capital invested and used in the provision of patient
care services by proprietary providers.

Supplemental Worksheet F consists of the following three parts:

        Part I   - Balance Sheet for Computation of Equity Capital
        Part II   - Computation of Return on Equity Capital of
                    Proprietary Providers
        Part III - Apportionment of Allowable Return on Equity
                    Capital of Proprietary Providers

385.1 Part I - Balance Sheet for Computation of Equity Capital.--
Proprietary providers are allowed a reasonable return on average
equity capital used to provide patient care. (See PRM, Part I,
chapter 12.)

Equity capital, as used in the health care programs, is the
owners' interest, subject to the prior claims of creditors, in
the provider organization or that part of such organization
rendering patient care. Equity capital is represented by the
excess of the assets related to patient care over the liabilities
related to patient care; the return allowed on such capital is
based on the health care programs' principles of reimbursement.
Equity capital must be computed for the health care complex as
a whole and the return must be allocated among the services
provided by each of the components of the health care complex
(e.g., hospital, subprovider, skilled nursing facility, home
health agency).

The first step in determining average equity capital during the
reporting period is to compute the amount of such capital at the
end of the accounting period. Supplemental Worksheet F, Part I,
is designed for this purpose. However, when a provider is
reporting for the first time under the health care programs, it
must complete Part I twice: once for the beginning of the cost
reporting period, and once for the end of the cost reporting
period. Part I should be completed through line 56 for the
beginning of the provider's first reporting period under the
health care programs. This is necessary so that the beginning
equity capital under the health care programs (see Part II,
column 2) can be determined.

At the end of the first reporting period under the health care
programs and in all subsequent reporting periods, Part I should
be completed through line 60. The ending equity capital
(line 56) will be transferred to Part II, column 8, on the line
representing the last month or period in the cost reporting
period. For example, if the cost report is for a 12-month
calendar year, this would be line 13 (December).

The ending equity capital (line 56) with adjustments (lines 57
through 59) will be the beginning equity capital for the
following period (line 60).

Columns 2 and 6--Enter the balances recorded in the provider's
books of account at the end of the reporting period. Attachments
may be used if the lines on the worksheet are not sufficient.

Columns 3 and 7--These columns are used to make any adjustments
to the amounts recorded in columns 2 and 6 that are required to
arrive at equity capital for Medicare cost reporting. Assets and
liabilities for renal dialysis equipment where the provider has
elected 100 percent reimbursement must be excluded. However, do
not make any adjustments to eliminate the assets and liabilities
applicable to a noncertified part of a skilled nursing facility
(see Worksheet A, line 53). These assets and liabilities should
remain in the total since the return on equity capital will be
apportioned over the entire health care complex. Some examples
of adjustments which may be required follow:

Line 1 - Cash on Hand and In Banks--Enter in column 3, the amount
of cash included in column 2 which is excessive and therefore
not needed for patient care services.

Funds deposited in a savings account for more than 6 consecutive
months are considered to have been diverted to income producing
activities which are not related to patient care.

Line 2 - Temporary Investments--Enter in column 3, the cost
applicable to temporary investments not related to patient care.

This item should be reduced by the amount, if any, that the investments as recorded in the books (column 2) exceed cost.

Lines 3 and 4 - Notes Receivable and Accounts Receivable--Enter in column 3, the notes and accounts receivable that are not for patient care services, but are included in the amounts recorded in column 2. This would include such items as balances due from owners, officers, employees, directors, stockholders and other miscellaneous sources.

Line 5 - Other Receivables--Enter in column 3, the amounts included in this receivable which did not result from patient care services. Normally, the total amount of this receivable would be entered in column 3.

Line 6 - Less: Allowance for Uncollectible Notes and Accounts Receivable--Enter in column 3, the amount of the allowance included in column 2 which is directly applicable to the amounts entered in column 3, lines 3, 4 and 5. The receivables on lines 3, 4 and 5 applicable to patient care services and includable in equity capital must reflect the amount that can reasonably be expected to be collected, regardless of the provider's method of computing bad debts.

Line 7 - Inventory--Enter in column 3, the cost of any inventory items which are not related to patient care. This includes, but is not limited to, the inventory cost of items applicable to the coffee shop and canteen. Also, include such items as replacement parts for television, etc., and other items related to noncovered services.

Line 8 - Prepaid Expenses--Enter any amounts in column 3 which are included in column 2, but are not related to patient care. This would include any items resulting from costs that are unallowable under the health care programs, such as prepaid premiums on life insurance carried by a provider on officers and key employees, where the provider is designated as the beneficiary.

Line 9 - Other Current Assets--Include in column 3, the full amount of any items in column 2 not related to patient care.

Lines 11, 12, 14, 16, 18, 20, 22, 24, 25 - Fixed Assets--Enter in column 3, the difference, if any, between the amounts entered in column 2 and the historical costs of the assets, or in the case of donated assets, the fair market value at the time of donation. Also, enter (1) the cost of any assets not related to patient care, and (2) the cost of any assets whose acquisition was determined not to be consistent with the standards, plans or criteria developed to meet the need for adequate health care facilities. (See PRM, Part I, chapter 24.)

Lines 13, 15, 17, 19, 21, 23 - Accumulated Depreciation and
Amortization--The amounts should be adjusted to reflect accumulated depreciation under the health care programs. Also, adjust
the accumulated depreciation and amortization in column 2 by
any amounts applicable to the related assets adjusted in
column 3.

Line 27 - Investments--Investments includable in equity capital
are limited to those related to patient care. Primarily, these
are temporary investments of operating funds (line 2). Operating
funds invested for long periods of time would be considered in
excess of patient care needs and should be deleted in column 3.
(See PRM, Part I, chapter 12.)

Line 28 - Deposits on Leases--Generally, deposits required under
the terms of a lease are included in equity capital. However,
enter in column 3, the cost of deposits for assets leased from
related organizations and for assets not related to patient
care. See the instructions for column 8, line 54, for the treatment of assets leased from related organizations. Also, enter
in column 3, any amount deposited under the terms of a lease or
comparable arrangement for any facility or part thereof or
equipment for a facility, the expenditures for which would have
been considered a capital expenditure and subject to exclusion
from reimbursement under titles V, XVIII and XIX had the provider
acquired it by purchase. (See PRM, Part I, chapter 24.)

Line 29 - Due From Owners/Officers--For adjustments to this
account, see instructions for lines 3, 4 and 5 above.

Line 30 - Special Funds--Gifts or grants which are unrestricted
as to use are includable in equity capital. However, funds which
are designated by other parties (grantors, donors, etc.) for
paying specific provider costs are not includable in equity
capital and the amount of such funds should be entered in column 3.

The amounts deposited in a funded depreciation account and the
earnings therefrom which remain in the fund are not includable
in equity capital and should be entered in column 3.

Line 31--This space is provided for other assets for which no
separate space is provided. An example of such assets is
deferred charges, which includes such items as Organization
Expense and Unamortized Bond Discount and Expense. These items
are properly included in equity capital if related to patient
care services.

Another example of such assets is goodwill. Goodwill purchased
in an acquisition prior to August 1970 of an existing organization is includable in the provider's equity capital. However,
goodwill which has not been purchased, but has been internally

generated as, for example, from a reorganization of the provider, is not includable in the provider's equity capital at any time.

For facilities or tangible assets acquired after July 1970, the excess of the purchase price paid for a facility or asset over (1) the historical cost of the tangible assets or (2) the cost basis of the tangible assets, whichever is applicable, is not includable in the computation of equity capital. (See PRM, Part I, chapter 12.)

A provider that is part of a chain operation may also include on this line its proportional share of the equity of its home office which is related to patient care. The equity in assets leased to members of a chain operation (or any organization which will use the equity in leased assets for Medicare reimbursement) must be excluded from the home office equity allocation, which is includable on line 31. See the instructions for line 54 concerning the treatment of equity in assets leased from related organizations. If the adjustment has not been made, the provider must adjust its share of home office equity to exclude the equity in such assets. (See PRM, Part I, chapter 21.)

Lines 34 through 50 - Liabilities--Enter in column 7, the amount of any liabilities which are directly attributable to and identifiable with the cost of any assets that were entered in column 3.

Lines 45 and 46 - Loans from Owners--Do not make adjustments in column 7 for funds borrowed prior to July 1, 1966, provided the terms and conditions of the loan agreement have not been modified subsequent to July 1, 1966. Such loans are considered as a liability in computing equity capital since interest expense related to such loans is included in allowable costs.

Where the terms and conditions of the loan agreement of loans made prior to July 1, 1966, have been modified subsequent to July 1, 1966, such loans are not included as a liability in column 8, and, therefore, should be adjusted in column 7. Loans from owners made after July 1, 1966, are not to be included as a liability in computing equity capital and should be adjusted in column 7.

Line 51 - Capital--The capital accounts in column 5, line 51, are those applicable to the type of business organizations under which the provider operates as follows:

       INDIVIDUAL PROPRIETOR - Proprietor's Capital Account
       PARTNERSHIP   - Partners' Capital Accounts
       CORPORATION   - Capital Stock and Other Accounts

Line 52 - Total Capital--Subtract the amount in column 7, line 50, from the amount in column 3, line 33, and enter the result on this line in column 7.

Columns 4 and 8--Adjust the amounts entered in columns 2 and 6 by the amounts (increase or decrease) entered in columns 3 and 7, and extend the net amounts to columns 4 and 8, respectively.

Line 52 - Total Capital--Subtract the amount in column 8, line 50, from the amount in column 4, line 33, and enter the result on this line in column 8.

Line 54 - Equity in Assets Leased From Related Organizations--If lease payments for real or personal property are not included in allowable cost because the lessor is a related organization as defined in the PRM, Part I, chapter 10, the owner's equity in the net cost of the leased assets is properly includable in equity capital. See the instructions for completing line 31. However, if the lease payments are included in allowable cost because of any of the exceptions cited in chapter 10, then the net value of the assets cannot be included in equity capital. The amount to be entered on line 54 is computed on the same basis as for assets owned directly by the provider organization. If the owner (related organization) has a negative equity in the assets leased to the provider, the negative amount rather than zero must be included on this line.

Line 55 - Difference Between Total Interim Payments and Net Cost of Covered Services--Enter the difference between total interim payments received and receivable for the cost reporting period and the net cost of covered services. The net cost of covered services used in this computation will not include the reimbursable return on equity capital. To obtain this difference enter the amount from Worksheet E, Part I, columns 1 through 8, line 26 plus Worksheet E, Part III, line 13 minus the amount from Worksheet E-1 (completed for each component of the health care complex) sum of categories 1 through 3, line 4. If the provider is claiming reimbursement from title V and/or title XIX in addition to title XVIII, also include in the amount entered on this line, the difference between the amount entered on Worksheet E-5, Part I, sum of columns 1 through 3, line 16, minus the amount received and receivable from intermediaries or State agencies for the current fiscal year on the accrual basis. The amount received and receivable from the intermediaries or State agencies must agree with the amount which will be entered on Worksheet E-5, Part III, sum of columns 1 through 3, line 10. A separate Worksheet E-5 for title V and title XIX must be completed and used in this computation.

If combined billing is being used, do not reduce the interim payments and the net cost of covered services for any amounts

applicable to the professional component of hospital-based
physicians. For purposes of this computation, it will be assumed
that these two amounts equal.

If the interim payments exceed the cost of covered services, the
amount constitutes a reduction of equity capital. If the interim
payments are less than the cost, add the difference to equity
capital. However, to the extent that the difference has already
been considered in this balance sheet, no entry should be made on
line 55.

Line 56 - Total Equity Capital--Enter the sum of line 52 plus/
minus lines 54 and 55. Enter negative amount in parenthesis
(   ).

        1. If line 56 is computed as of the end of the cost
reporting period and the amount computed on line 56 is a positive
or negative amount, transfer this amount to Part II, column 8,
for the last month or period in the cost reporting period.

        2. If line 56 is computed as of the beginning of a cost
reporting period (first reporting period under the health care
programs only) and the amount computed on line 56 is a positive
or negative amount, transfer this amount to Part II, column 2,
all lines, and column 8, line 1.

The balance of this worksheet provides for adjusting equity
capital for the beginning of the following cost reporting period.
Do not complete lines 57-60 until the cost report has been
completed for the current period.

Line 57 - Return on Equity Capital--Enter on this line the amount
of reimbursable return on equity capital computed in Part III.

The amount to be entered is the sum of the following from Part III:

        1. The return on equity capital in column 3 for all
provider components on lines 4 and 6;

        2. The return on equity capital in column 3, line 5
(Part A only) and the return on equity capital in column 4b,
line 5 (Part B only) for those provider components whose reasonable cost on Worksheet E, Part II, the sum of the Part A and
Part B columns, line 5, is less than customary charges on
Worksheet E, Part II, sum of the Part A and Part B columns, line 20;
and/or

        3. The return on equity capital in column 3, line 5
(Part A and Part B) for those provider components whose customary
charges on Worksheet E, Part II, sum of the Part A and Part B
columns, line 20, are less than reasonable cost on Worksheet E,
Part II, sum of the Part A and Part B columns, line 5.

Line 58 - Adjustments to Health Care Program Costs--The total equity capital entered on line 56 should be adjusted to reflect any increases or decreases which may be needed to properly reflect the beginning equity for the subsequent cost reporting period. Some adjustments to be considered in this computation are:

    1. A decrease by the amount of the excess reasonable cost over customary charges (sum of amounts entered on Worksheet E, Part II, columns 1 through 8, line 24, and Worksheet E-5, Part II, columns 1 through 3, line 17), and

    2. An increase by the amount of the recovery of unreimbursed costs from prior cost reporting periods (sum of amounts entered on Worksheet E, Part III, columns 1, 3, 5 and 7, lines 10 and 11, columns 2, 4, 6 and 8, line 12; and Worksheet E-5, Part III, columns 1 through 3, lines 5 and 6.

Line 59 - Federal, State and Local Income Taxes--For purposes of determining the amount of equity capital at the end of the reporting period, corporate providers and noncorporate providers taxed as corporations will accrue their income tax liability prior to the determination of the reimbursable return on equity capital, the cost limitations adjustments and reimbursable bad debts. The amount of this liability should be entered in column 8, line 40.

After reimbursable return on equity capital, bad debts and the computation of any adjustments entered on line 58 have been determined, any income taxes attributable to these amounts should be entered on line 59.

Line 60 - Total Equity Capital Beginning of Following Cost Reporting Period--Enter on this line the sum of lines 56 and 57, plus or minus lines 58 and 59. This total, whether positive or negative, is the beginning equity capital for the following cost reporting period and will be shown in Part II, column 2, all lines and in column 8, line 1.

385.2 Part II - Computation of Return on Equity Capital of Proprietary Providers.--This part provides for the computation of the average equity capital and the amount of return includable in allowable costs.

Column 1--List each of the months or periods included in the cost reporting period.

Column 2--Enter the equity capital as of the beginning of the cost reporting period, as computed on the previous year's Worksheet F, Part I, column 8, line 60 (line 56 if first reporting period under the health care programs). This amount will be the same for all months or periods during the cost reporting period. Also, enter this amount in column 8, line 1.

Column 3--List by month or period the capital investments made during the cost reporting period. Capital investments include cash and other property contributed by owners and proceeds from the issuance of corporate stocks. Do not include loans from owners here. The amount entered on the appropriate line in column 3 is carried forward to subsequent months in the period, and is increased by additional contributions in the month(s) or period(s) in which such contributions are made.

Column 4--Enter the net gain or loss from the disposition of depreciable assets computed in accordance with the PRM, Part I, chapter 1. Gains and losses on investments related to patient care and included in equity capital will also be shown in this column.

Beginning with the month or period in which the transaction occurs, the amount of gain or loss is carried forward to subsequent months or periods in the cost reporting period and is increased or decreased as further asset disposals occur.

Column 5--Enter in this column the amounts withdrawn by owners or disbursed for the personal benefit of owners; any amounts paid as dividends to corporate stockholders are also entered. This column includes the cumulative amount for the period; i.e., if withdrawals occur at the rate of $600 per month or period, the first month or period of the cost reporting period will show $600, the second - $1,200, etc. However, if withdrawals are made and are reflected in the profit or loss for the period (for example, as salaries), they should not be entered here.

Column 6--Enter other changes in equity capital such as loans from owners made after July 1, 1966 (increases) and repayments of the same (decreases). Unrestricted donations and contributions are also entered in this column. Beginning with the first month or period in which a transaction occurs, the applicable amount is carried forward to subsequent months or periods and is increased by additional loans or decreased by repayments of loans.

Column 7--Equity capital increases or decreases as income is earned or as losses are incurred in operations of the provider during the cost reporting period.

The net amount of the change in equity capital that results from operations is determined by analyzing the difference between equity capital at the beginning of the period and equity capital at the end of the period. From this increase or decrease in equity capital are added or subtracted the amounts included under the other categories of changes on this worksheet,

columns 3 through 6. The balance then will represent the increase
or decrease due to operations.

To compute the increase or decrease due to operations for the last
month or period within the cost reporting period (if the cost
report is for a 12-month calendar year, this would be line 13 -
December) subtract from the ending equity capital (from Part I,
line 56), which should be entered on line 13, column 8, the total
of columns 2 through 6 (same line). If the amount in Part I,
line 56, is negative, use the negative amount for this computation.
Enter the resulting amount in column 7 (same line). This increase
or decrease due to operations is considered to have been experienced
uniformly during each of the months or periods of the cost
reporting period and to have affected equity cumulatively. Therefore, if the net increase due to profits for 12 months is $24,000
(as entered in column 7, line 13), there would be $2,000 entered
on line 2, $4,000 entered on line 3, etc.

Column 8--For each month or period within the cost reporting
period, enter the net total of columns 2 through 7. The amount
shown will be the actual amount, whether positive or negative.

Column 9--Where the provider includes a distribution of equity
capital from a home office (or other related organization), enter
the monthly amounts of equity capital allocated from the home
office (or other related organization) whether positive or negative.
The amounts entered in this column must equal the provider's
portion of the home office (or other related organization) equity
capital from form HCFA-2552G, Supplemental Worksheet F, Part II,
column 8, or from a similar worksheet. See PRM, Part I,
chapters 12 and 21.

Column 10--The provider equity capital and allocated home office
(or other related organization) equity capital will be combined
in this column. If the combined equity capital in any month is
a negative amount, a zero should be shown for that month.

If the provider is not associated with a home office (or other
related organization), the amounts in column 8 will be brought
forward to column 10 and when the equity capital in any month is
a negative amount, a zero should be shown for that month.

Add the individual months' equity capital and enter the total of
column 10 on line 15.

Line 16 - Computation of Return on Equity Capital--Divide the
total amount shown in column 10, line 15, by the number of months
or periods in the cost reporting period plus one to determine
average equity capital during the period. If this is a short
period report, make this computation as stated in the previous
line and an adjustment will be made on line 17. Apply the

appropriate rate of return to the average equity capital to determine the amount of return includable in allowable costs. The
intermediary will furnish the rate of return.

Line 17--The amount computed on line 16 will yield the allowable
return for a full year. If a shorter reporting period is
covered by this worksheet, the full year return must be divided
by the number of months (12) or periods that would otherwise be
contained in a full reporting period. This resulting amount will
then be multiplied by the number of months or periods included in
the worksheet to arrive at the amount of return to be included in
allowable costs. Enter this amount on line 17.

385.3 Part III - Apportionment of Allowable Return on Equity
Capital of Proprietary Providers.--This worksheet provides for
the apportionment of the allowable return on equity capital to
the various health care programs. The method of apportionment is
based on the ratio of the allowable return on equity capital
(line 1) to total allowable costs (line 2). This ratio (line 3)
is applied to the health care program costs entered in column 2,
lines 4a through 6c. References for obtaining the appropriate
health care program costs (column 2) are listed in column 1.

Note the references for obtaining the amount to be entered on
line 2. If a provider received a grant, etc., which was offset on
Worksheet A-8, line 59, and such grant was applicable to a revenue
producing cost center and exceeded the total direct costs and
overhead allocations after cost finding (i.e., the cost center
reflected a credit balance on Worksheet B, column 21) the amount
of such credit balance should be added to the amount to be entered
on line 2.

The allowable return on equity capital entered in column 3, line 4
(title V) and line 6 (title XIX) is transferred to Worksheet E-5,
Part II, column as appropriate, line 3. The allowable return on
equity capital applicable to title XVIII (column 3, lines 5a through
5h) is transferred to Worksheet E, Part II, columns 1-8, as
appropriate, line 3. The allowable return on equity capital applicable to title XVIII (column 3, lines 5i through 5k) is transferred
to form HCFA-1728A. These amounts are needed for the computation
of the lesser of reasonable cost or customary charges.

The amounts in column 3, lines 5b, 5d, 5f, 5h and 5k applicable to
title XVIII - Part B must be multiplied by 80 percent in column 4
to determine reimbursable amounts. On line 5j, enter in column 4b
the same amount entered in column 3.

The reimbursable return on equity capital applicable to title XVIII -
Part A (column 3, lines 5a, 5c, 5e and 5g) and the amount applicable to title XVIII - Part B (column 4b, lines 5b, 5d, 5f and
5h) is transferred to Worksheet E, Part III, columns 1-8, as
appropriate, line 2.

390.   SUPPLEMENTAL WORKSHEET A-8-3 - REASONABLE COST DETERMINATION
       FOR PHYSICAL THERAPY SERVICES FURNISHED BY OUTSIDE SUPPLIERS
This worksheet provides for the computation of any needed
adjustments to costs applicable to physical therapy services furnished by outside suppliers. The information required on this
worksheet must provide for, in the aggregate, all data for physical
therapy services furnished by all outside suppliers in determining
the reasonableness of the physical therapy costs. (See PRM,
Part I, chapter 14.)

390.1 Part I - General Information.--This part provides for
furnishing certain information concerning physical therapy services
furnished by outside suppliers.

Lines 1a-1d--Enter on these lines by type of employee the total
hours of service for all patients. For services performed at the
provider site, enter the total number of hours by each type of
employee physically present during the reporting period. (To
define supervisors, see PRM, Part I, chapter 14.) The hours shown
should reflect the activities of all the outside suppliers excluding
travel time to and from the provider. Do not include any time for
employees of the provider.

For home health services performed at the patient's residence,
enter the number of hours physically present at the patient's residence, excluding travel time. If time records are not available,
one visit equals 1 hour.

Line 2--This calculation is used to determine whether services are
full time or intermittent part time. For services performed at
the provider site, count only those weeks during which a supervisor,
therapist or an assistant was onsite. For services performed at
the patient's residence, count only those weeks during which
services were rendered by supervisors, therapists, or assistants
to patients of the home health agency. Weeks where services were
performed both at the provider's site and at the patient's home
are only counted once. (See PRM, Part I, chapter 14.)

Line 3--Enter amounts paid and/or payable to the outside supplier
for services rendered during the reporting period as reported in
the cost report. This includes any payments for supplies, equipment use, overtime or any other expenses.

Where the provider furnishes physical therapy services by outside
suppliers for health care program patients, but simply arranges
for such services for nonhealth care program patients and does not
pay the nonhealth care program portion of such services, its books
will reflect only the cost of the health care program portion.
Where the provider can "gross up" its costs in accorance with
provisions of the PRM, Part I, chapter 23, it will complete lines 9
or 10, as appropriate, and the costs on this line must be "grossed

up." See the instructions on Worksheet C with respect to "grossing up" of the provider's charges. However, where the provider cannot "gross up" its costs, it must complete line 10 only.

390.2 Part II - Travel Allowance/Expense Computation.--This part provides for the computation of the standard travel allowance and expense. The optional travel allowance computation may only be used for home health patient services if time records are available. Since the rates to be used in the computation may change during the provider's cost reporting period, the lines are separated into two parts to show the periods affected by the change in rates. (See PRM, Part I, chapter 14, or latest publication of rates to be used in the computation.)

Lines 5a-5e--These lines provide for the computation of the standard travel allowance/expense for physical therapy services performed at the provider site.

One standard travel allowance is recognized for each day an outside supplier performs skilled services at the provider site. For example, if a contracting organization sends three therapists to a provider each day, only one travel allowance is recognized per day.

Lines 6a-6e--These lines provide for the computation of the standard travel allowance/expense for physical therapy services performed in conjunction with home health agency visits. These lines will only be used if the provider does not opt for the optional method of computing travel on line 7. A standard travel allowance is recognized for each visit to a patient's residence. If services are furnished to more than one patient at the same location, only one standard travel allowance is permitted, regardless of the number of patients treated.

Lines 7a-7k--These lines provide for the optional travel allowance/expense computation for therapy services in conjunction with home health services only. (See PRM, Part I, chapter 14.) Lines 7a-7e will be used for computing the optional travel allowance and lines 7f-7j will be used for computing the optional travel expense.

390.3 Part III - Salary Equivalent Computation.--This part provides for the computation of the full-time or intermittent part-time salary equivalency.

Since the hourly rate allowances to be used in the computation may change during the provider's cost reporting period, the lines are separated into two parts to show the periods affected by the change in rates. (See PRM, Part I, chapter 14, or latest publication of allowable hourly rates for therapists to be used in the computation on lines 9a and 9c, and 10b and 10f.)

The cost of services of a therapy aide or trainee will be
evaluated at an hourly rate not to exceed the hourly rate paid to
the provider's employees of comparable classification and/or qualification, e.g., nurses' aides. The cost of the services of a
physical therapy assistant will be evaluated at the going hourly
rate paid by providers in the area to salaried physical therapy
assistants. The 50 percent fringe benefit and expense factor will
then be added to the hourly rate determined appropriate for therapy
assistants, aides and trainees. If the going hourly rate for
physical therapy assistants in the area is unobtainable, the
physical therapy assistants' compensation may be evaluated at a
rate not to exceed three quarters of the hourly salary equivalency
amount. Since this amount includes the 50 percent fringe benefit
and expense factor, no further adjustment to the amount would be
needed.

Lines 9a-9e--These lines are to be completed for the salary
equivalency computation only when line 2 of Part I is greater
than the sum of lines la-lc of Part I. The reasonable cost of
intermittent, part-time services may not exceed the amount which
would be allowable had the provider purchased the services on a
regular part-time basis for an average of 15 hours per week. The
hours of service for aides are not included in this determination,
but the cost of their services will be included in the overall
cost determination.

The hourly rate allowance amounts entered in column 2, lines 9a
and 9c, will be the therapist hourly rate allowance amounts. The
sum of the therapist hours to be entered in column 1, lines 9a and
9c must equal line 2.

The sum of the aide hours to be entered in column 1, lines 9b and
9d must equal line 1d.

Lines 10a-10i--These lines are to be completed for the salary
equivalency computation only when line 2 of Part I is less than
the sum of lines la-lc of Part I. The limitation for the cost of
these services will be based on the reasonableness of cost of
full-time or regular part-time services. The hours of service
for aides are not included in this determination, but the cost
of their services will be considered in the cost determination
based on actual number of hours worked. The sum of the hours
entered in column 1 must equal the sum of the hours on lines la
through 1d.

390.4 Part IV - Overtime Computation.--This part provides for the
computation of an overtime allowance when an individual employee
of the outside supplier performs services for the provider in
excess of the provider's standard workweek. No overtime allowance
may be given to a therapist who receives an additional allowance
for supervisory or administrative duties.

Since the rates to be used in the computation may change during the
provider's cost reporting period, this part is set up to facilitate the periods affected by the change in rates. (See PRM, Part I,
chapter 14, or latest publication of allowable hourly rates for
therapists to be used in the computation for lines 12, 18, 24 and
30.)

The cost of services of a therapy aide or trainee will be
evaluated at an hourly rate not to exceed the hourly rate paid to
the provider's employees of comparable classification and/or
qualification, e.g., nurses' aides. The cost of the services of
a physical therapy assistant will be evaluated at the going hourly
rate paid by providers in the area to salaried physical therapy
assistants. The 50 percent fringe benefit and expense factor will
then be added to the hourly rate determined appropriate for therapy
assistants, aides and trainees.

If the going hourly rate for physical therapy assistants in the
area is unobtainable, the physical therapy assistants' compensation
may be evaluated at a rate not to exceed three quarters of the
hourly salary equivalency amount. Since this amount includes the
50 percent fringe benefit and expense factor, no further adjustment to the amount would be needed.

Lines 11 and/or 23--Enter in the appropriate column for each
period the total overtime hours worked. The sum of the hours on
lines 11 and 23 is entered in column 4 of line 23.

Lines 12 and/or 24--Enter in the appropriate column for each
period the overtime rate which is the hourly rate allowance times
1.5.

Lines 15 and/or 27--Enter the percentage of overtime hours by
class of employee which is determined by dividing each column on
lines 11 and 23 by the total overtime hours in column 4, line 23.

Lines 16 and/or 28--These lines are for the allocation of a
provider's standard workyear for one full-time employee. Enter
the standard workyear for one full-time employee in column 4,
line 28. Multiply the standard workyear in column 4, line 28,
by the percentages on lines 15 and 27 and enter the results in
the corresponding column on lines 16 and 28.

Lines 18 and/or 30--Enter in the appropriate column the hourly
rate allowance for each class of employee for each period.

390.5 Part V - Limitation Computation.--This part provides for
the calculation of the adjustment to physical therapy service
costs in determining the reasonableness of cost.

Lines 39 and 40--Where the outside supplier provides the equipment
and supplies used in furnishing direct services to the provider's
patients, the actual costs of the equipment and supplies incurred
by the outside supplier, as specified in PRM, Part I, chapter 14,
may be considered in the total allowed cost.

399. EXHIBITS

   A. Worksheets.--

Exhibit 1 - Worksheet Checklist

Exhibit 2 - Hospital, Hospital-Skilled Nursing Facility Complex
               and Skilled Nursing Facility Statistical Data -
               Part I

Exhibit 3 - Hospital, Hospital-Skilled Nursing Facility Complex
               and Skilled Nursing Facility Statistical Data -
               Parts II and III

Exhibit 4 - Hospital, Hospital-Skilled Nursing Facility Complex
               and Skilled Nursing Facility Statistical Data -
               Parts IV and V

Exhibit 5 - Worksheet A

Exhibit 6 - Worksheet A-1

Exhibit 7 - Worksheet A-2

Exhibit 8 - Worksheets A-3, A-4 and A-5

Exhibit 9 - Worksheet A-6

Exhibit 10 - Worksheet A-7

Exhibit 11 - Worksheet A-8

Exhibit 12 - Worksheets A-8-1 and A-8-2

Exhibit 13 - Worksheet B

Exhibit 14 - Worksheet B-1

Exhibit 15 - Worksheet C

Exhibit 16 - Worksheet D

Exhibit 17 - Worksheet D-1, Part I

Exhibit 18 - Worksheet D-1, Part II

Exhibit 19 - Worksheet D-2

Exhibit 20 - Worksheet D-3

Exhibit 21 - Worksheet D-8

Exhibit 22 - Worksheet E, Part I

Exhibit 23 - Worksheet E, Part II

8-80   FORM HCFA-2552   399(Cont.)

Exhibit 24 - Worksheet E, Part III

Exhibit 25 - Worksheet E-1

Exhibit 26 - Worksheet E-2

Exhibit 27 - Worksheet E-5, Parts I and II

Exhibit 28 - Worksheet E-5, Part III

Exhibit 29 - Worksheet G

Exhibit 30 - Worksheet G-1

Exhibit 31 - Worksheet G-2

Exhibit 32 - Worksheet G-3

    B. <u>Supplemental Worksheets (Available Upon Request From Intermediary)</u>.--

Exhibit S-1   -   HCFA-2552A - Supplemental Worksheets D-4 and D-5

Exhibit S-2   -   HCFA-2552B - Supplemental Worksheet D-6

Exhibit S-3   -   HCFA-2552C - Supplemental Worksheet D-7

Exhibit S-4   -   HCFA-2552D - Supplemental Worksheet E-3

Exhibit S-5   -   HCFA-2552E - Supplemental Worksheet E-4

Exhibit S-6   -   HCFA-2552F - Supplemental Worksheet E-4-1

Exhibit S-7   -   HCFA-2552G - Supplemental Worksheet F, Part I

Exhibit S-8   -   HCFA-2552G - Supplemental Worksheet F, Part II

Exhibit S-9   -   HCFA-2552G - Supplemental Worksheet F, Part III

Exhibit S-10 -   HCFA-2552H - Supplemental Worksheet A-8-3,
                                  Parts I, II and III

Exhibit S-11 -   HCFA-2552H - Supplemental Worksheet A-8-3,
                                  Parts IV and V

Exhibit 1

Form Approved
OMB No. 66-R0078

**WORKSHEET CHECKLIST FOR HOSPITAL, HOSPITAL-SKILLED NURSING FACILITY
COMPLEX AND SKILLED NURSING FACILITY COST REPORT**

PROVIDER NO: _____

PERIOD: FROM _____ TO _____

| CHECK THE APPROPRIATE COLUMN FOR EACH WORKSHEET | Completed | | Not Applicable |
	HCFA Worksheet	Substitute Worksheet	
WORKSHEETS	1	2	3
1 Worksheet Checklist			
2 Hospital and Hospital-Skilled Nursing Facility Complex and Skilled Nursing Facility Statistical Data – Part I			
3 Hospital and Hospital-Skilled Nursing Facility Complex and Skilled Nursing Facility Statistical Data – Parts II and III			
4 Hospital and Hospital-Skilled Nursing Facility Complex and Skilled Nursing Facility Statistical Data – Parts IV and V			
5 Worksheet A			
6 Worksheet A-1			
7 Worksheet A-2			
8 Worksheet A-3			
9 Worksheet A-4			
10 Worksheet A-5			
11 Worksheet A-6			
12 Worksheet A-7			
13 Worksheet A-8			
14 Worksheet A-8-1			
15 Worksheet A-8-2			
16 Worksheet B			
17 Worksheet B-1			
18 Worksheet C			
19 Worksheet D			
20 Worksheet D-1 – Part I (All Pages Must Be Completed)			▓▓▓▓▓
21 Worksheet D-1 – Part II			
22 Worksheet D-2			
23 Worksheet D-3			
24 Worksheet D-8			
25 Worksheet E – Part I			
26 Worksheet E – Part II			
27 Worksheet E – Part III			
28 Worksheet E-1			
29 Worksheet E-2			
30 Worksheet E-5 – Parts I and II			
31 Worksheet E-5 – Part III			
32 Worksheet G			
33 Worksheet G-1			
34 Worksheet G-2			
35 Worksheet G-3			
SUPPLEMENTAL WORKSHEETS (AVAILABLE UPON REQUEST FROM INTEMEDIARY):			
36 HCFA-2552A – Supplemental Worksheet D-4			
37 HCFA-2552A – Supplemental Worksheet D-5			
38 HCFA-2552B – Supplemental Worksheet D-6			
39 HCFA-2552C – Supplemental Worksheet D-7			
40 HCFA-2552D – Supplemental Worksheet E-3			
41 HCFA-2552E – Supplemental Worksheet E-4			
42 HCFA-2552F – Supplemental Worksheet E-4-1			
43 HCFA-2552G – Supplemental Worksheet F – Part I			
44 HCFA-2552G – Supplemental Worksheet F – Part II			
45 HCFA-2552G – Supplemental Worksheet F – Part III			
46 HCFA-2552H – Supplemental Worksheet A-8-3			

If substitute worksheets are a part or all of this cost report (a check in column 2), enter the name and address of the person, company or forms preparation service which originated the substitute worksheets:

NAME : _____

ADDRESS: _____

_____

Form HCFA-2552 (5-80)
Destroy old stock

Exhibit 2

This report is required by law (42 USC 1395g; 20 CFR 405.406[b]) Failure to report can result in all interim payments made since the beginning of the cost report period being deemed overpayments (42 USC 1395g).

Form Approved
OMB No. 56-R0078

HOSPITAL, HOSPITAL-SKILLED NURSING FACILITY COMPLEX AND SKILLED NURSING FACILITY STATISTICAL DATA	INTERMEDIARY USE ONLY	DATE RECEIVED
	☐ AUDITED ☐ DESK REVIEWED	INTERMEDIARY NO.

PART I – GENERAL

1. Names and Addresses	Provider Numbers	Dates Certified
HOSPITAL		
SUBPROVIDER I		
SUBPROVIDER II		
SKILLED NURSING FACILITY		
HOME HEALTH AGENCY		
SPECIAL PROVIDER-CONTROLLED FACILITY		

2. Cost Reporting Period	From	TO

3. Type of Control

a. Voluntary Nonprofit
- ☐ Church
- ☐ Other *(Specify)*

b. Proprietary
- ☐ Individual
- ☐ Corporation
- ☐ Partnership
- ☐ Other *(Specify)*

c. Government
- ☐ Federal
- ☐ City-County
- ☐ County
- ☐ State
- ☐ Hospital District
- ☐ City
- ☐ Other *(Specify)*

4. Type of Hospital

a.
- ☐ General-Short Term
- ☐ General-Long Term
- ☐ Tuberculosis
- ☐ Specialty Short-Term
- ☐ Specialty Long-Term
- ☐ Chronic Disease
- ☐ Psychiatric
- ☐ Other *(Specify)*

b. Medicare Certified
Kidney Transplant Hospital   ☐ Yes   ☐ No

5. Type of Skilled Nursing Facility
- ☐ Entirely Certified Skilled Nursing Facility
- ☐ Partially Certified Skilled Nursing Facility
- ☐ Skilled Nursing Facility Unit of Domiciliary Institution
- ☐ Skilled Nursing Facility Unit of Rehabilitation Center
- ☐ Other *(Specify)*

6. Health Care Programs   ☐ Title V   ☐ Title XVIII   ☐ Title XIX

7.
a. Are management and/or administrative support services purchased from an outside supplier or organization?   ☐ Yes ☐ No
b. If yes, what is the total amount for these services included on Worksheet A, column 7? $

INTENTIONAL MISREPRESENTATION OR FALSIFICATION OF ANY INFORMATION CONTAINED IN THIS COST REPORT MAY BE PUNISHABLE BY FINE AND/OR IMPRISONMENT UNDER FEDERAL LAW

CERTIFICATION BY OFFICER OR ADMINISTRATOR OF PROVIDER(S)

I HEREBY CERTIFY that I have read the above statement and that I have examined the accompanying Statement of Reimbursable Cost and the Balance Sheet and Statement of Revenue and Expense prepared by _____

(Provider name[s] and number[s]) for the cost report period beginning _____ and ending

_____ , and that to the best of my knowledge and belief, it is a true, correct, and complete statement prepared from the books and records of the provider(s) in accordance with applicable instructions, except as noted.

(Signed) _____
Officer or Administrator of Provider(s)

Title _____

Date _____

Form HCFA-2552 (5-80)

2

Exhibit 3

Form Approved
OMB No. 98-R0078

HOSPITAL, HOSPITAL-SKILLED NURSING FACILITY COMPLEX AND SKILLED NURSING FACILITY STATISTICAL DATA	PROVIDER NO.:	PERIOD: FROM _____ TO _____

PART II – HOSPITAL STATISTICS

	INPATIENT – ALL PATIENTS	GENERAL SERVICE	SPECIAL CARE UNITS			
			ICU	CCU	OTHER (SPECIFY)	
		1	2	3	4	5
1	Beds (excluding newborn) available at beginning of period					
2	Beds (excluding newborn) available at end of period					
3	Total bed days available (excluding newborn)					
4	Aged, pediatric and maternity inpatient days					
5	Other than aged, pediatric and maternity inpatient days (excl. newborn)					
6	Total inpatient days (excluding newborn) (Sum of lines 4 and 5)					
7	Percent occupancy (line 6 ÷ line 3)	%	%	%	%	%
8	Total newborn inpatient days					
	INPATIENT – HEALTH CARE PROGRAMS					
9	TITLE V					
	a. Inpatient days (excluding newborn)					
	b. Newborn inpatient days					
10	TITLE XVIII					
	a. Aged, pediatric and maternity inpatient days (excluding kidney acquisition days)					
	b. Kidney acquisition days (aged, pediatric and maternity)					
	c. Total aged, pediatric and maternity inpatient days (Sum of lines 10a and 10b)					
	d. Other than aged, pediatric and maternity inpatient days (excluding kidney acquisition days)					
	e. Kidney acquisition days (other than aged, pediatric and maternity)					
	f. Total other than aged, pediatric and maternity inpatient days (Sum of lines 10d and 10e)					
	g. Total inpatient days (excluding kidney acquisition days) (Sum of lines 10c and 10d)					
	h. Total kidney acquisition days (Sum of lines 10b and 10e)					
	i. Total Part A inpatient days (Sum of lines 10g and 10h)					
	j. Total Part B inpatient days (SEE INSTRUCTIONS)					
	k. Part B inpatient days when Part A benefits are not available (SEE INSTRUCTIONS)					
11	TITLE XIX					
	a. Inpatient days (excluding newborn)					
	b. Newborn inpatient days					

	OUTPATIENT – HEALTH CARE PROGRAMS	TITLE V	TITLE XVIII	TITLE XIX	ALL OTHER	TOTAL (SUM OF COLS 1-4)
12	Number of occasions of service (exclusive of renal dialysis treatments)					

PART III – OTHER HOSPITAL DATA

1	Amount of accelerated payments outstanding as of end of cost reporting period – title XVIII	$
2	Average number of employees on payroll for the period (full-time equivalent) – excludes nonpaid workers	
3	Average number of nonpaid workers for the period (full-time equivalent) for which reimbursement is claimed	
4	Number of renal dialysis treatments (inpatient and outpatient)	
	a. Total – All Hospital Patients	
	b. Title V	
	c. Title XVIII	
	d. Title XIX	
5	Number of admissions (excluding newborn)	
	a. Total – All Hospital Inpatients	
	b. Title V	
	c. Title XVIII	
	d. Title XIX	
6	Number of discharges including deaths (excluding newborn)	
	a. Total – All Hospital Inpatients	
	b. Title V	
	c. Title XVIII	
	d. Title XIX	
7	Average length of stay	
	a. Total (Part II, line 6 [sum of cols 1-5] ÷ Part III, line 6a)	
	b. Title V (Part II, line 9a [sum of cols 1-5] ÷ Part III, line 6b)	
	c. Title XVIII (Part II, line 10i [sum of cols 1-5] ÷ Part III, line 6c)	
	d. Title XIX (Part II, line 11a [sum of cols 1-5] ÷ Part III, line 6d)	

Exhibit 24

FORM APPROVED
OMB NO. 0938-0050

CALCULATION OF REIMBURSEMENT SETTLEMENT—TITLE XVIII
PART A AND PART B SERVICES

PROVIDER NO.	PERIOD: FROM ___ TO ___	WORKSHEET E PART I

PART I — COMPUTATION OF NET COST OF MEDICARE-COVERED SERVICES

DESCRIPTION	HOSPITAL			SUBPROVIDER I		SUBPROVIDER II		SKILLED NURSING FACILITY		
	PART A	PART B 100%	PART B 80%	PART A	PART B	PART A	PART B	PART A	PART B	
	1	2	3	4	5	6	7	8	9	
1 Inpatient ancillary services (From Wkst D, cols 7 & 8, line 28)	$		$	$	$	$	$	$	$	1
2 Outpatient services (SEE INSTRUCTIONS)		$								2
3 Inpatient routine services (From Wkst D-1, Part 1, line 43)										3
4 Intern and resident services (From Wkst D-2, Part 1[cols 9-10, Part II, col 5, or Part III, col 6, as appropriate)										4
5 Utilization review-physicians' compensation (From provider records)										5
6 Hospital-based pathologists remuneration—SNF inpatients (From Supplemental Wkst D-4, line 5)										6
7 Ambulance services (From Supplemental Wkst D-5, col 2, line 5)										7
8 Kidney acquisition costs-supplementary to inpatient routine & inpatient ancillary service costs (From Supplemental Wkst D-6, Part I, line 7)										8
9 Cost of service furn. "under arrangements" to Medicare beneficiaries only										9
10 Malpractice insurance costs (From Wkst D-8, Parts II and IV, as approp.)										10
11 Services of Teaching Physicians (SEE INSTRUCTIONS)										11
12 SUBTOTAL (Sum of lines 1-11)	$	$	$	$	$	$	$	$	$	12
13 Differential in charges between semiprivate accommodations and less than semiprivate accommodations	( )		( )	( )		( )		( )		13
14 Total kidney acquisition charges billed to Medicare under Part B (From provider records)	( )		( )	( )		( )		( )		14
15 SUBTOTAL (Part A—line 12 minus sum of lines 13 and 14) (Part B—sum of lines 12 and 14)	$	$	$	$	$	$	$	$	$	15
16 Amounts paid and payable by Workers' Compensation	( )		( )	( )		( )		( )		16
17 Total revenue received for kidneys furnished to other providers, kidney procurement organizations, and others and for kidneys transplanted in non-Medicare patients (From provider records)	( )		( )	( )		( )		( )		17
18 SUBTOTAL (Part A—line 15 minus sum of lines 16 & 17) (Part B—from line 15)	$	$	$	$	$	$	$	$	$	18
19 Part A deductibles and coinsurance billed to Medicare patients	( )		( )	( )		( )		( )		19
20 Bad debts for deductibles and coinsurance, net of bad debt recoveries	( )		( )	( )		( )		( )		20
21 Net deductibles and coinsurance billed to Medicare patients (line 19 minus 20)										21
22 Net Cost of Medicare-covered services, excluding return on equity capital and adjustment for Part B costs (Part A—line 18 minus line 21) (Part B—from line 18)	$	$	$	$	$	$	$	$	$	22

33

Exhibit 25

FORM APPROVED
OMB NO. 0938–0050

CALCULATION OF REIMBURSEMENT SETTLEMENT—TITLE XVIII PART A AND PART B SERVICES	PROVIDER NO.:	PERIOD: FROM ______ TO ______	WORKSHEET E PART II

PART II — COMPUTATION OF THE LESSER OF REASONABLE COST OR CUSTOMARY CHARGES

	DESCRIPTION	HOSPITAL PART A 1	HOSPITAL PART B 100% 2	HOSPITAL PART B 80% 3	SUBPROVIDER I PART A 4	SUBPROVIDER I PART B 5	SUBPROVIDER II PART A 6	SUBPROVIDER II PART B 7	SKILLED NURSING FACILITY PART A 8	SKILLED NURSING FACILITY PART B 9	
23	Reasonable cost of title XVIII—Part A and Part B services										23
24	Cost of services (From Part I, line 15)	$	$	$	$	$	$	$	$	$	24
25	Allowable return on equity capital (From Supp. Wkst. F, Part III, col. 3, line 5)										25
26	Renal dialysis cost in excess of limitation (From Supp. Wkst. E-3, sum of cols. 1–3, line 11)			( )						( )	26
27	TOTAL reasonable cost of title XVIII—Part A and Part B services (Sum of lines 24 & 25 minus line 25)	$	$	$	$	$	$	$	$	$	27
28	Charges for title XVIII—Part A and Part B services										28
29	Inpatient ancillary services (SEE INSTRUCTIONS)										29
30	Outpatient services (SEE INSTRUCTIONS)										30
31	Inpatient routine services (From provider records)										31
32	Intern and resident services (From provider records)										32
33	Ambulance services (From Supp. Wkst. D-5, col. 1, line 5)										33
34	Kidney acquisition charges-supplementary to inpatient routine and inpatient ancillary service charges (From Supp. Wkst. D-6, Part II, line 4)										34
35	Charges for serv. furnished "under arrang'mts" to Medicare beneficiaries only										35
36	Total kidney acq. charges billed to Medicare under Part B	( )			( )		( )				36
37	Services of Teaching Physicians (From Provider Records)										37
38	Total charges for title XVIII—Part A & Part B services (Sum of lines 29–37)	$	$	$	$	$	$	$	$	$	38
39	Customary charges										39
40	Aggregate amount actually collected from patients liable for payment for services on a charge basis	$			$		$		$		40
41	Amounts that would have been realized from patients liable for payment for service on a charge basis had such payment been made in accordance with Health Insurance Regulation 405.455(b)	$			$		$		$		41
42	Ratio of line 40 to line 41 (not to exceed 1.00000000)										42
43	TOTAL customary charges (line 38 × line 42)	$	$	$	$	$	$	$	$	$	43
44	Excess of aggregate charges over aggregate cost (Sum of cols., line 43 minus sum of columns, line 27) (Complete line 46)	$			$		$		$		44
45	Excess of aggregate cost over aggregate charges (Sum of columns, line 27 minus sum of columns, line 43) (Complete line 47)	$			$		$		$		45
46	Excess of customary charges over reasonable cost (Complete only if line 43 exceeds line 27) (Enter lesser of line 43 minus line 27 or line 44) (Transfer to Supp. Wkst. E-4, Part I, line 1)	$	$	$	$	$	$	$	$	$	46
47	Excess of reasonable cost over customary charges (Complete only if line 27 exceeds line 43) (Enter lesser of line 27 minus line 43 or line 45) (Transfer to Supp. Wkst. E-4, Part III, line 3b)	$	$	$	$	$	$	$	$	$	47

FORM HCFA–2552–81 (11–81)

34

Exhibit 26

FORM APPROVED
OMB NO. 0938-0050

CALCULATION OF REIMBURSEMENT SETTLEMENT—TITLE XVIII
PART A AND PART B SERVICES

PROVIDER NO. _____

PERIOD:
FROM _____
TO _____

WORKSHEET E
PART III

PART III — COMPUTATION OF REIMBURSEMENT SETTLEMENT

DESCRIPTION	HOSPITAL			SUBPROVIDER I		SUBPROVIDER II		SKILLED NURSING FACILITY	
	PART A	PART B 100%	PART B 80%	PART A	PART B	PART A	PART B	PART A	PART B
	1	2	3	4	5	6	7	8	9
48 Cost of Medicare covered services including return on equity capital (Part A & Part B—100%—Sum of lines 22 & 25) (Part B—80%—From line 27)									48
49 Part B deductibles billed to Medicare patients (excludes coinsurance amounts)									49
50 Part B deductibles billed to Medicare patients (excludes coinsurance amounts)									50
51 Excess reasonable cost (From line 47)									51
52 SUBTOTAL (Line 50 minus 51)									52
53 80% of Part B costs (line 52 × 80%)									53
54 Part B coinsurance billed to Medicare patients (From provider record)									54
55 Net cost Part B for comparison (line 52 minus line 54)									55
56 Reimbursable bad debts (SEE INSTRUCTIONS)									56
57 Inpatient professional services rendered by hospital-based radiologists & pathologists (SEE INSTRUCTIONS)									57
58 Inpatient professional services rendered by hospital-based radiologists & pathologists (SEE INSTRUCTIONS)									58
59 Outpatient professional services rendered by hospital-based physicians (SEE INSTRUCTIONS)									59
60 Outpatient professional services rendered by hospital-based physicians (SEE INSTRUCTIONS)									60
61 TOTAL COST—Current cost reporting period (Part A, line 52) (Part B—100%, line 52 plus line 56 thru 60) (Part B—80%, lesser of line 53 or line 55 plus lines 56 thru 60)									61
62 Recovery of unreimbursed costs under lesser of cost or charges (From Supp. Wkst. E-4, Part II, line 2)									62
63 Recovery of unreimbursed costs under lesser of cost or charges (From Supp. Wkst. E-4, Part III, cols. 1, 2 and 3, line 2e)									63
64 80% of recovery of unreimbursed cost under lesser of cost or charges (line 63)—Part B									64
65 Home Program Dialysis Equipment—100% Medicare (From Wkst. B, col. 21, line 88)									65
66 Amounts applicable to prior cost reporting periods resulting from disposition of depreciable assets									66
67 Recovery of excess depreciation resulting from provider termination or a decrease in Medicare utilization									67
68 Unrefunded charges to beneficiaries for excess costs erroneously collected, based on correction of cost limit									68
69 TOTAL COST reimbursable to provider (Part A—sum of lines 61-63 plus/minus line 66 minus sum of lines 67-68) (Part B—100%—sum of lines 61 and 63 plus/minus lines 65-66) (Part B—80%—sum of lines 61 and 64 plus/minus line 66 minus line 67)									69
70 Interim payments (From Wkst E-1, line 4)									70
71 Carrier payments (From provider records)									71
72 TOTAL payments (Sum of lines 70 and 71)									72
73 Balance due provider/Medicare (line 69 minus line 72) (indicate overpayment in brackets)									73

FORM HCFA-2552-81 (11-81)

35

Exhibit 27

FORM APPROVED
OMB NO. 0938-0050

ANALYSIS OF PAYMENTS TO PROVIDERS FOR SERVICES RENDERED TO TITLE XVIII (MEDICARE) BENEFICIARIES

WORKSHEET E-1

PROVIDER NO.

PERIOD: FROM — TO —

CHECK ONE: ☐ HOSPITAL ☐ SUBPROVIDER I ☐ SUBPROVIDER II ☐ SKILLED NURSING FACILITY

DESCRIPTION		CATEGORY 1 INPATIENT PART A		CATEGORY 2 INPATIENT PART B		CATEGORY 3 OUTPATIENT PART B/100%		CATEGORY 4 OUTPATIENT PART B/80%	
		MO/DAY/YR	AMOUNT	MO/DAY/YR	AMOUNT	MO/DAY/YR	AMOUNT	MO/DAY/YR	AMOUNT

1 Total interim payments paid to provider

2 Interim payments payable on individual bills, either submitted or to be submitted to the intermediary for services rendered in the cost reporting period. If none, write "NONE."

3 List separately each retroactive lump sum adjustment amount based on subsequent revision of the interim rate for the cost reporting period. Also show date of each payment. If none, write "NONE."
   Program to Provider (a, b, c, d, e)
   Provider to Program (f, g, h, i, j)

SUBTOTAL (sum of lines 3a–3e minus sum of lines 3f–3j) (k)

4 TOTAL INTERIM PAYMENTS (sum of lines 1, 2, and 3k) (Transfer to Wkst. E, Part III, col. as appropriate, line 70)

TO BE COMPLETED BY INTERMEDIARY

5 List separately each tentative settlement payment after desk review. Show date of each payment. If none, write "NONE."
   Program to Provider (a, b, c, d, e)
   Provider to Program (f)

SUBTOTAL (sum of lines 5a–5c minus sum of lines 5d–5f) (g)

6 Determined net settlement amount (balance due) based on the cost report (1)
   Program to Provider (a)
   Provider to Program (b)

7 TOTAL MEDICARE PROGRAM LIABILITY (Reimbursable cost, net of deductibles and coinsurance) (line 4 plus/minus lines 5g and 6) (Should equal amounts entered on Wkst. E, Part III, col. as appropriate, line 69)

NAME OF INTERMEDIARY | INTERMEDIARY NUMBER | SIGNATURE OF AUTHORIZED PERSON | DATE (MO/DAY/YR)

(1) On lines 3, 5 and 6, where an amount is due "Provider to Program," show the amount and date on which the provider agrees to the amount of repayment, even though total repayment is not accomplished until a later date.

FORM HCFA-2552-81 (11-81)

36

Exhibit 28

FORM APPROVED
OMB NO. 0938-0050

CALCULATION OF REIMBURSEMENT SETTLEMENT ☐ TITLE V ☐ TITLE XIX	PROVIDER NO.:	PERIOD: FROM _____ TO _____	WORKSHEET E-5 PART I & II

PART I — COMPUTATION OF NET COST OF COVERED SERVICES

	DESCRIPTION	HOSPITAL 1	SUBPROVIDER I 2	SUBPROVIDER II 3
1	Inpatient ancillary services (From Wkst. D, col. 6 or 9, line 28)	$	$	$
2	Inpatient routine services (From Wkst. D-1, Part II, line 67)			
3	Intern and resident services (From Wkst. D-2, Part I, col. 8 or 10, lines 9, 10, and 11)			
4	Ambulance Services (From Supplemental Wkst. D-5, col. 2, line 4 or 6)		░░░░░░░	░░░░░░░
5	Malpractice insurance costs (From Worksheet D-8, Parts II and III, as appropriate)			
6	Kidney acquisition costs (SEE INSTRUCTIONS)			
7	Services of Teaching Physicians (From Supp. Wkst. D-9, line 3, col. 5a or 5g)			
8	SUBTOTAL (Sum of lines 1–7)	$	$	$
9	Differential in charges between semiprivate accommodations and less than semiprivate accommodations	( )	( )	( )
10	SUBTOTAL (line 8 minus line 9)	$	$	$
11	Inpatient professional services rendered by hospital-based physicians (For title V—from Wkst. D-3, Part I, col. 5a, line 12 plus Part II, col. 5a, line 12) (For title XIX—from Wkst. D-3, Part I, col. 5f, line 12 plus Part II, col. 5g line 12)			
12	Amounts paid and payable by Worker's Compensation	( )	( )	( )
13	SUBTOTAL (Sum of lines 10 and 11 minus line 12)	$	$	$
14	Deductibles and coinsurance billed to health care program inpatients	$	$	$
15	Bad debts for deductibles and coinsurance, net of bad debt recoveries.	( )	( )	( )
16	Net deductibles and coinsurance billed to health care program inpatients (line 14 minus line 15)	$	$	$
17	Net cost of covered services to health care program inpatients, excluding return on equity capital (line 13 minus line 16)	$	$	$

PART II — COMPUTATION OF LESSER OF REASONABLE COST OR CUSTOMARY CHARGES

	DESCRIPTION	HOSPITAL 1	SUBPROVIDER I 2	SUBPROVIDER II 3
18	Reasonable cost of inpatient services	░░░░░░░	░░░░░░░	░░░░░░░
19	Cost of services (From Part I, line 10)	$	$	$
20	Allowable return on equity capital (From Supplemental Wkst. F, Part III, line 4 or line 6)			
21	TOTAL reasonable cost of inpatient services (Sum of lines 19 and 20)	$	$	$
22	Charges for inpatient services	░░░░░░░	░░░░░░░	░░░░░░░
23	Inpatient ancillary services (SEE INSTRUCTIONS)	$	$	$
24	Inpatient routine services (From provider records)			
25	Ambulance services (From Supplemental Wkst. D-5, col. 1, line 4 or 6)			
26	Services of Teaching Physicians (From Provider Records)			
27	TOTAL charges for inpatient services (Sum of lines 23–26)	$	$	$
28	Customary charges	░░░░░░░	░░░░░░░	░░░░░░░
29	Aggregate amount actually collected from patients liable for payment for services on a charge basis (From provider records)	$	$	$
30	Amounts that would have been realized from patients liable for payment for services on a charge basis had such payment been made in accordance with Health Insurance Reg. Sec. 405.455(b) (From provider records)	$	$	$
31	Ratio of line 29 to line 30 (Not to exceed 1.00000000)			
32	TOTAL customary charges (line 27 × line 31)	$	$	$
33	Excess of customary charges over reasonable cost (line 32 minus line 21) (Transfer to Supplemental Wkst. E-4, Part I, line 1, col. 1)	$	$	$
34	Excess of reasonable cost over customary charges (line 21 minus line 32) (Transfer to Supplemental Wkst. E-4, Part III, line 3b)	$	$	$

Rev. 15   3-191

Exhibit 29

FORM APPROVED
OMB NO. 0938-0050

CALCULATION OF REIMBURSEMENT SETTLEMENT ☐ TITLE V ☐ TITLE XIX	PROVIDER NO.:	PERIOD: FROM _____ TO _____	WORKSHEET E-5 PART III

PART III — COMPUTATION OF REIMBURSEMENT SETTLEMENT

	DESCRIPTION	HOSPITAL	SUBPROVIDER I	SUBPROVIDER II
		1	2	3
35	Net cost of covered services to health care program inpatients, excluding return on equity capital (From Part I, line 17)	$	$	$
36	Reimbursable return on equity capital (From Part II, line 20)			
37	SUBTOTAL (Sum of lines 35 and 36)	$	$	$
38	Excess reasonable cost (From Part II, line 34)	( )	( )	( )
39	Recovery of unreimbursed costs under cost limits (From Supplemental Wkst E-4, Part II, line 2)			
40	Recovery of unreimbursed costs under lesser of cost or charges (From Supplemental Wkst. E-4, Part III, col. 1, line 2e)			
41	Amounts applicable to prior cost reporting periods resulting from disposition of depreciable assets			
42	Recovery of excess depreciation resulting from provider termination or a decrease in Medicare utilization	( )	( )	( )
43	TOTAL COST—reimbursable to provider (Sum of lines 37, 39 and 40 minus sum of lines 38 and 42 plus or minus line 41)	$	$	$
44	Amount received and receivable from intermediary or State agency for current fiscal year on accrual basis (Exclude accelerated payments; include lump sum interim payments)	( )	( )	( )
45	Carrier payments (From provider records)	( )	( )	( )
46	Total payments (Sum of lines 44 and 45)	( )	( )	( )
47	Balance due provider/health care program (line 43 minus line 46) (Indicate overpayment in brackets)	$	$	$

Exhibit 30

FORM APPROVED
OMB NO. 0938-0050

WORKSHEET G

BALANCE SHEET

(To be completed by all providers maintaining fund type accounting records. Nonproprietary providers not maintaining fund type accounting records, should complete the "General Fund" column only)

PROVIDER NO.: _____

PERIOD: FROM ___ TO ___

	ASSETS (Omit Cents)	GENERAL FUND	SPECIFIC PURPOSE FUND	ENDOWMENT FUND	PLANT FUND
	CURRENT ASSETS				
1.	Cash on hand and in banks	$	$	$	$
2.	Temporary Investments				
3.	Notes Receivable				
4.	Accounts Receivable				
5.	Other Receivables				
6.	Less Allowance for uncollectible notes and accounts receivable	( )	( )	( )	( )
7.	Inventory				
8.	Prepaid Expenses				
9.	Other Current Assets				
10.	Due From Other Funds				
11.	TOTAL CURRENT ASSETS (Sum of lines 1–10)	$	$	$	$
	FIXED ASSETS				
12.	Land	$	$	$	$
13.	Land Improvements				
14.	Less Accumulated Depreciation	( )	( )	( )	( )
15.	Buildings				
16.	Less Accumulated Depreciation	( )	( )	( )	( )
17.	Leasehold Improvements				
18.	Less Accumulated Amortization	( )	( )	( )	( )
19.	Fixed Equipment				
20.	Less Accumulated Depreciation	( )	( )	( )	( )
21.	Automobile & Trucks				
22.	Less Accumulated Depreciation	( )	( )	( )	( )
23.	Major Movable Equipment				
24.	Less Accumulated Depreciation	( )	( )	( )	( )
25.	Minor Equipment Nondepreciable				
26.	Other Fixed Assets				
27.	TOTAL FIXED ASSETS (Sum of lines 12–26)	$	$	$	$
	OTHER ASSETS				
28.	Investments	$	$	$	$
29.	Deposits on leases				
30.	Due from owners/officers				
31.					
32.	TOTAL OTHER ASSETS (Sum of lines 28–31)	$	$	$	$
33.	TOTAL ASSETS (Sum of lines 11, 27, & 32)	$	$	$	$

	LIABILITIES AND FUND BALANCES (OMIT CENTS)	GENERAL FUND	SPECIFIC PURPOSE FUND	ENDOWMENT FUND	PLANT FUND
	CURRENT LIABILITIES				
34.	Accounts Payable	$	$	$	$
35.	Salaries, Wages & Fees Payable				
36.	Payroll Taxes Payable				
37.	Notes & Loans Payable (Short Term)				
38.	Deferred Income				
39.	Accelerated Payments				
40.	Due to Other Funds				
41.					
42.	TOTAL CURRENT LIABILITIES (Sum of lines 34–41)	$	$	$	$
	LONG-TERM LIABILITIES				
43.	Mortgage Payable	$	$	$	$
44.	Notes Payable				
45.	Unsecured Loans				
46.	Loans from owners — a. Prior to 7/1/66 / b. On or after 7/1/66				
47.					
48.					
49.	TOTAL LONG-TERM LIABILITIES (Sum of lines 43–48)	$	$	$	$
50.	TOTAL LIABILITIES (Sum of lines 42 & 49)	$	$	$	$
	CAPITAL ACCOUNTS				
51.	General Fund Balance	$	$	$	$
52.	Specific Purpose Fund Balance				
53.	Donor created—Endowment Fund Balance—Restricted				
54.	Donor created—Endowment Fund Balance—Unrestricted				
55.	Governing Board created—Endowment Fund Balance				
56.	Plant Fund Balance—Invested in Plant				
57.	Plant Fund Balance—Reserve for Plant Improvement, Replacement and Expansion				
58.	TOTAL FUND BALANCES (Sum of lines 51 thru 57)	$	$	$	$
59.	TOTAL LIABILITIES AND FUND BALANCES (Sum of lines 50 & 58)	$	$	$	$

( ) = contra amount

39

Exhibit 31

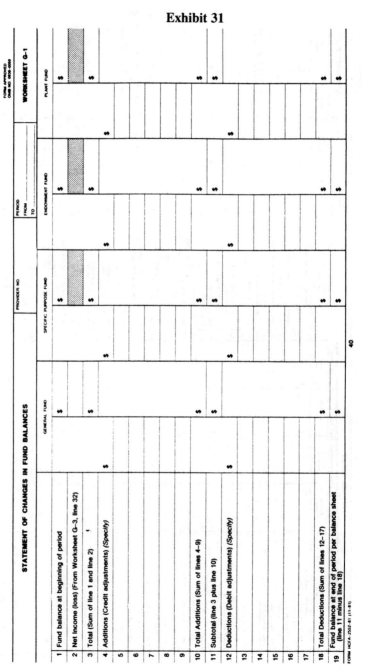

Exhibit 32

FORM APPROVED
OMB NO. 0938-0050

STATEMENT OF PATIENT REVENUES AND OPERATING EXPENSES	PROVIDER NO.:	PERIOD: FROM _____ TO _____	WORKSHEET G-2

PART I - PATIENT REVENUES

	REVENUE CENTER	INPATIENT 1	OUTPATIENT 2	TOTAL 3
1	GENERAL INPATIENT ROUTINE CARE SERVICE			
2	Hospital	$		$
3	Subprovider I			
4	Subprovider II			
5	Skilled Nursing Facility—Certified			
6	Skilled Nursing Facility—Noncertified			
7	TOTAL General Inpatient Routine Care Service (Sum of lines 2–6)	$		$
8	SPECIAL INPATIENT CARE SERVICE			
9	Intensive Care Unit	$		$
10	Coronary Care Unit			
11				
12				
13	TOTAL Special Care Service (Sum of lines 9–12)	$		$
14	TOTAL Inpatient Routine Care Service (Sum of lines 7 & 13)	$		$
15	Ancillary Service		$	
16	Outpatient Service			
17	Home Health Agency			
18	Ambulance			
19				
20				
21	TOTAL Patient Revenues (Sum of lines 14–20) (Transfer col. 3 to WKST G-3, line 1)	$	$	$

PART II - OPERATING EXPENSES

1 Operating Expenses (Per Worksheet A, col. 3, line 84).. $ _____

2 Add (Specify).. $ _____

3 .... _____

4 .... _____

5 .... _____

6 .... _____

7 .... _____

8 TOTAL Additions (Sum of lines 2–7).. _____

9 Deduct (Specify).. $ _____

10 .... _____

11 .... _____

12 .... _____

13 .... _____

14 TOTAL Deductions (Sum of lines 9–13).. (_____)

15 TOTAL Operating Expenses (Sum of lines 1 and 8 minus line 14) (Transfer to Worksheet G-3, line 4).. $ _____

FORM HCFA-2552-81 (11-81)   41

Exhibit 33

FORM APPROVED
OMB NO. 0938-0050

STATEMENT OF REVENUE AND EXPENSES	PROVIDER NO.:	PERIOD: FROM _____ TO _____	WORKSHEET G-3

1	Total patient revenues (From Wkst G-2, Part 1, col 3, line 21)	$ _____
2	Less-Allowances and discounts on patients' accounts	_____
3	Net patient revenues (line 1 minus line 2)	$ _____
4	Less-Total operating expenses (From Wkst G-2, Part II, line 15)	_____
5	Net income from serice to patients (line 3 minus line 4)	$ _____
6	Other income:	
7	Contributions, donations, bequests, etc. .... $ _____	
8	Income from investments	_____
9	Revenue from telephone and telegraph service	_____
10	Revenue from television and radio service	_____
11	Purchase discounts	_____
12	Rebates and refunds of expenses	_____
13	Parking lot receipts	_____
14	Revenue from laundry and linen service	_____
15	Revenue from meals sold to employees and guests	_____
16	Revenue from rental of living quarters	_____
17	Revenue from sale of medical and surgical supplies to other than patients	_____
18	Revenue from sale of drugs to other than patients	_____
19	Revenue from sale of medical records and abstracts	_____
20	Tuition (Fees, sale of textbooks, uniforms, etc.)	_____
21	Revenue from gifts, flower, coffee shops, and canteen	_____
22	Revenue from vending machines	_____
23	Rental of hospital space	_____
24	Other (Specify)	_____
25	Other (Specify)	_____
26	Total other income (Sum of lines 7-25)	_____
27	Total (line 5 plus line 26)	$ _____
28	Other expenses (Specify) .... $ _____	
29	....	_____
30	....	_____
31	Total other expenses (Sum of lines 28-30)	_____
32	Net income (or loss) for the period (line 27 minus line 31)	$ ========

FORM HCFA-2552-81 (11-81)

42

Index

About the Author

DONALD F. BECK, M.B.A., C.P.A., is one of America's foremost authorities on hospital finance. After a very successful career as a hospital financial officer, Mr. Beck started his own consulting firm, D. F. Beck & Associates, headquartered in Memphis.

Mr. Beck is the author of *Basic Hospital Financial Management,* a favorite reference as well as a widely used textbook. He serves on the editorial board and is a frequent contributor to *The Health Care Supervisor*; is on the editorial board and writes a financial feature for *Hospital Topics*; and writes a health care economics/financial feature for *Southern Hospitals.*

In addition to a busy consulting schedule, Mr. Beck has presented over 100 seminars, has appeared on television shows as an expert on hospital costs, and is in demand as a public speaker. Using his extensive experience in both the for-profit and the not-for-profit sectors, Mr. Beck has successfully generated hundreds of thousands of additional dollars for hospitals throughout the United States.